Let it pop!
JJ HUDSON

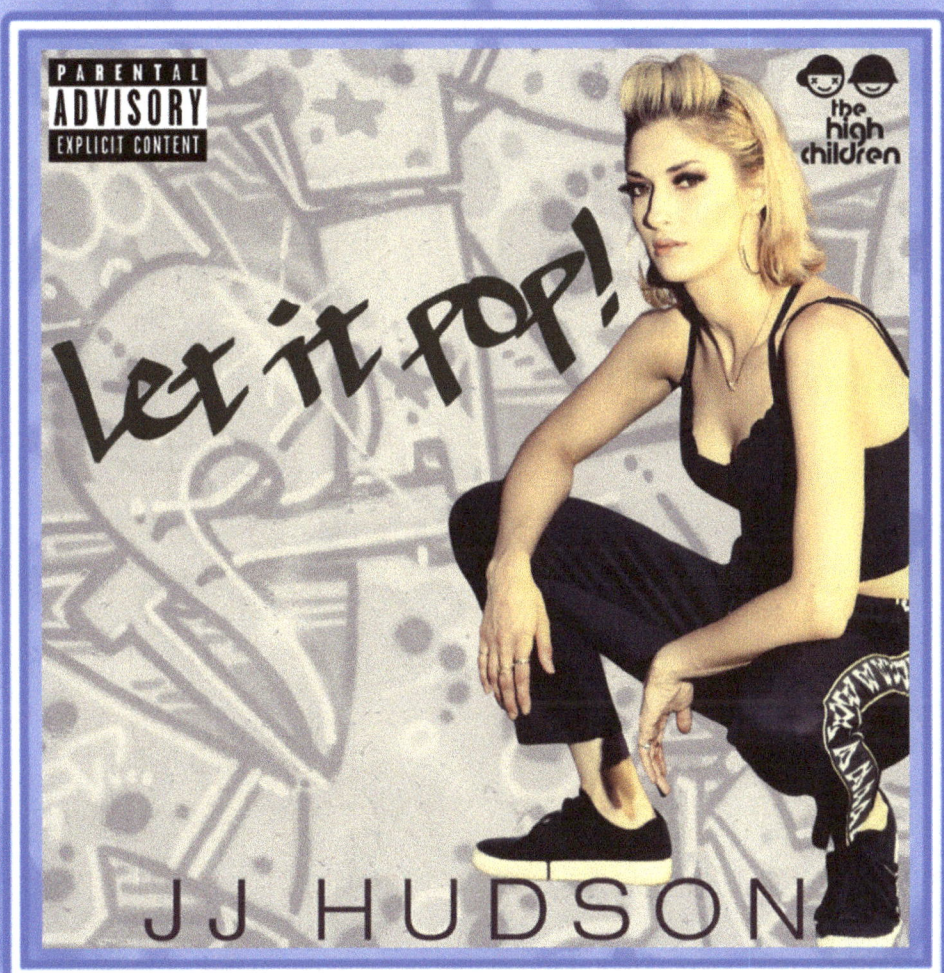

IN STORES NOW

Pump it up Magazine

TABLE OF CONTENTS

⚡ **THE HIGH CHILDREN**
JJ HUDSON - GRANDMIXER GMS - DJ NASTY NES
are back with a smash! "Let It Pop"

⚡ **EDITORIAL** 6
Page 5

⚡ **MASKS DOWN SMILING FACES!**
- Get Ready To Dance! Best Music Festivals 2021
- 5 Fun Outdoor Workouts For Summer
- Top Indie Artists
- Books: Mandalas Colouring Book For Children
- My Test(imony) by Paulette Jackson

⚡ **REVIEW** 11
Make Music With The Power Of Your Mind With Next Mind - Oculus Quest 2

⚡ **STYLE**
- Hit The Beach With Style!

⚡ **BEAUTY** 26
- Natural Beauty Tips You Will Love!

⚡ **MUST WATCH**
Summer of Soul

⚡ **TOP TIPS** 30
Make A Living With Your Music

⚡ **HUMANITARIAN AWARENESS**
World Environment Day

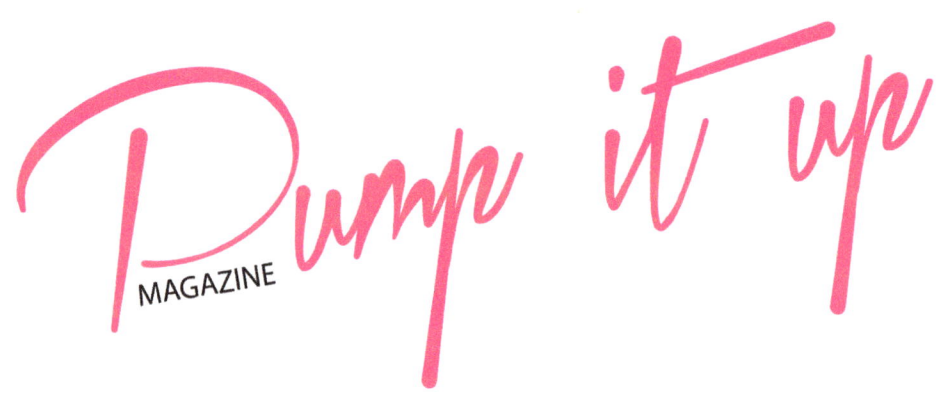

PUMP IT UP MAGAZINE
LINKS

WEBSITE
www.pumpitupmagazine.com

FACEBOOK
www.facebook.com/pumpitupmagazine

TWITTER
www.twitter.com/pumpitupmag

SOUNDCLOUD
www.soundcloud.com/pumpitupmagazine

INSTAGRAM
pumpitupmagazine

PINTEREST
www.pinterest.com/pumpitupmagazine

PUMP IT UP MAGAZINE
30721 Russell Ranch Road
Suite 140
Westlake Village,
California 91362
United States
www.pumpitupmagazine.com
info@pumpitupmagazine.com
Tel : (001) (877)841 – 7414 (toll free number)

EDITORIAL

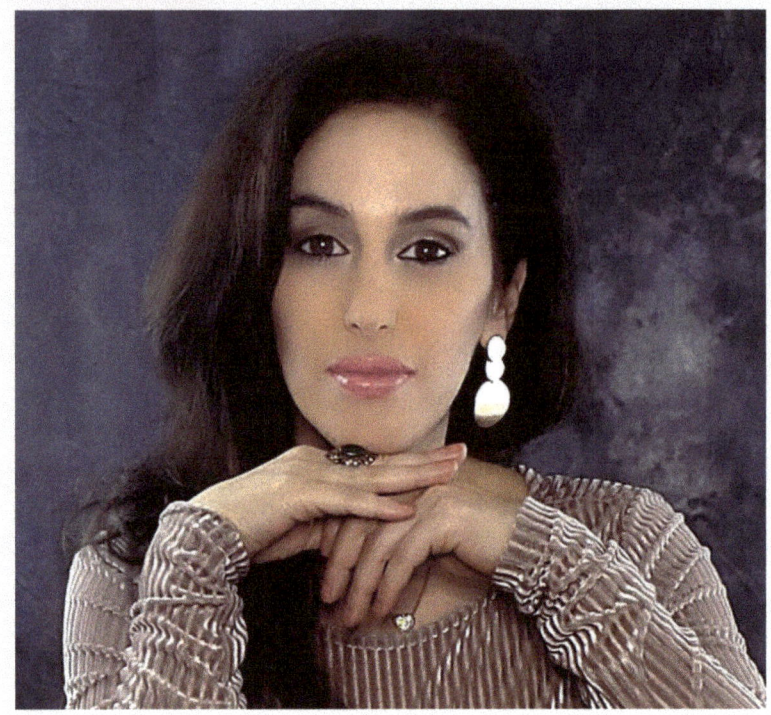

Greetings Readers,

June is here and summer is right around the corner

And its Black Music Month.

On the cover is the hot hip hop group High Children

Their new single is slammin Let It Pop!

Check them out!

Masks are off and we can now see smiling faces that we've missed for over a year.

Stadiums and concert halls are starting to fill up. So are we heading back to some form of normalcy? I sure hope so !

Inside the magazine we have a great article that depicts the future of listening to music via Oculus Qwest

We're talking controlling virtual reality with your mind!

Become fit and in shape for the summer with tips on keeping your body moving.

And there is more , but you will have to open and read to more goodies.

Tune in to Pump It Up Magazine Radio. It's your go to station for the best in hip hop/pop/r&b/soul, Jazz and more!

So stay cool, it's about to get hot!

Anissa Boudjaoui

CONTRIBUTORS

EDITOR IN CHIEF
Anissa Boudjaoui

MUSIC
Michael B. Sutton
A. Scott Galloway
Sarah Kaye

FASHION
Tiffani Sutton

MARKETING
Grace Rose

PARTNERS

Editions L.A.
www.editions-la.com

The Sound Of L.A.
www.thesoundofla.com

Info Music
www.infomusic.fr

Delit Face
www.DelitFace.com

L.A. Unlimited
www.launlimitedinc.com

**Photo Credits
The High Children
Teresa Felzer
Ian Phares
Jerry Hoo.**

THE HIGH CHILDREN

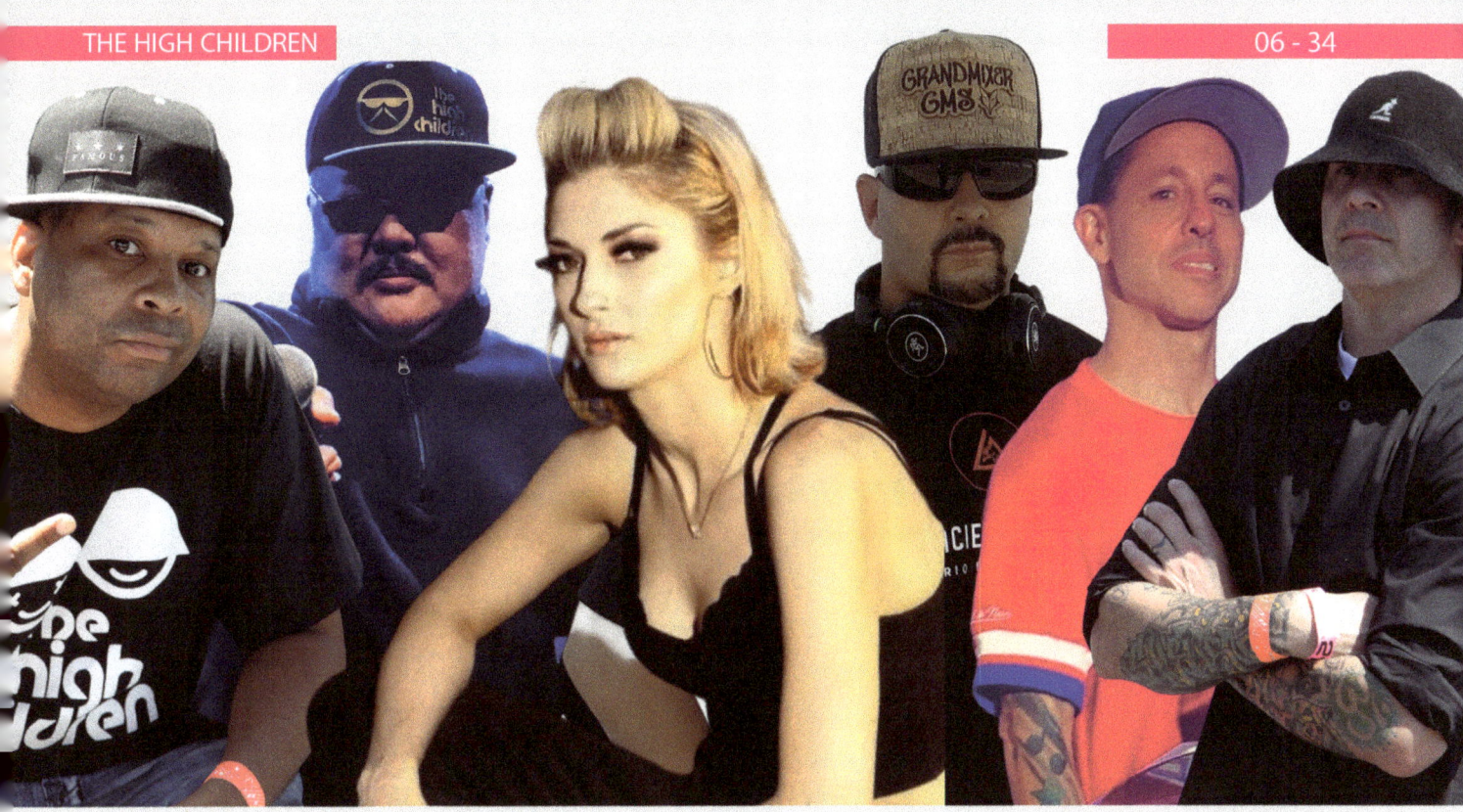

The High Children (photo from left to right) contains Jamal, DJ Nasty Nes, JJ Hudson, GrandMixer GMS, Dj Third Degree, Jayson, as members. Originating in the early 2000s became an instant hit with their positive energy being the message behind their music. Their melodic singing coupled with the rap styled catchy hooks along with their LIVE on-stage rap performances made them widely desired at the Seattle hip-hop scene and had them playing on MPC's, SP1200's, and turntables.

The Chief Evangelist, DJ Nasty Nes has been on the Seattle hip-hop scene for 41 Nes debuted the West Coast's first ever all rap radio show "Freshtracks" on Seattle's 1250 KFOX in 1980. Freshtracks was a two hour show that played on Sunday nights on KKFX 1250 ("KFOX") and consisted of a mix of new songs and a master mix created by Nasty Nes. *Nastymix Records, the Northwest's first hip-hop label, was founded in 1985 with the local release of Sir Mix-A-Lot's "Square Dance Rap". Nasty Nes is the guy who actually discovered Sir Mix-A-Lot.* Nastymix Records gained international recognition with *Sir Mix-A-Lot's 1992 #1 hit, "Baby Got Back"(year end Billboard chart #4, though on Def American Records). In 1988, Nes took his rap radio show 'Rap Attack' to KCMU and his 'Hotmix' show to KUBE 93.* Nes moved to South California in 1997 to became the rap editor for HITS magazine and five years later established rapattacklives.com, his own online promotions business. In 2019, DJ Nasty Nes revived his classic radio show, KFOX Nightbeat, featuring songs he originally played on Fresh Tracks and Nightbeat, as well as exclusive new music, and master mixes by GrandMixer GMS. Nes, in his own words said,

"Seeing Grandmaster Flash perform live on the wheels in New York gave me the incentive to be a radio DJ and a mix DJ"

GrandMixer GMS first hit the spotlight as a break-dancer at 11 years old and then in 1986, became the 1st DJ to mix for commercial radio in Spokane at just 14 years of age. GMS won the Inland Northwest Battle of the DJ's and began mixing with Tobin Costen on Spokane's then only all rap show in 1993. After these successful accolades, GMS began mixing for Nasty-Nes on Seattle's KCMU Rap Attack till he retired from music in the mid 90's.

THE HIGH CHILDREN

JJ Hudson, aka Jmoji, is the VP Fashion of the High Children brand. The talented artist's single "J", topped the charts on the latest top 30 college rap radio hits. JJ Hudson's hit single "J" was remixed by Nes & GMS.

The High Children brand has evolved itself into a brand embodying all: their music, fashion, and entertainment with video being the predominant language of their art form.

Jayson Ramos, CEO of The High Children brand is currently the head of video at Amazon Web Services, providing solutions to the multi-billion dollar company leveraging his music production, writing and performance experience.

The High Children brand's CIO, Jamal Allen has been the music host on Canada's MTV Select. He has produced remixes for Snoop dog, Mike Jones, Ashley Tisdale and Blake Lewis while working as an instructor for AT&T and DEV Tech as well.

Peter Maroda, CXO of the High Children brand introduced digital production to the record label Nastymix Records in the 90's. He has also managed a creative service agency providing services to Microsoft, Getty Images and Nordstrom. At Amazon, he grew an account and project management team with a focus on leveraging new processes, tools and data, increasing operational scale over 10x.

VP Promotions of the High Children brand Tim Jaffe has been a DJ since 12 years of age and has been involved in the music industry for the last 35 years now. He has been a host, music producer and DJ for several brands over the years. Tim Jaffe, DJ 3rd Degree, authors a weekly review column of new music for www.rapattacklives.com and is the host for Hot For The Streets Drive Time Mix Show (Wednesdays at 8pm EST/5pm PST) & The Coast to Coast Hip Hop Show (Fridays at 8pm EST/5pm PST) on www.EsWayRadio.com.

Robbie Rob is the VP Music Operations at the High Children brand.
Website: WWW.THEHIGHCHILDREN.COM

The High Children brand envisions itself having fun, staying young, inspired and taking its goals to the highest level!

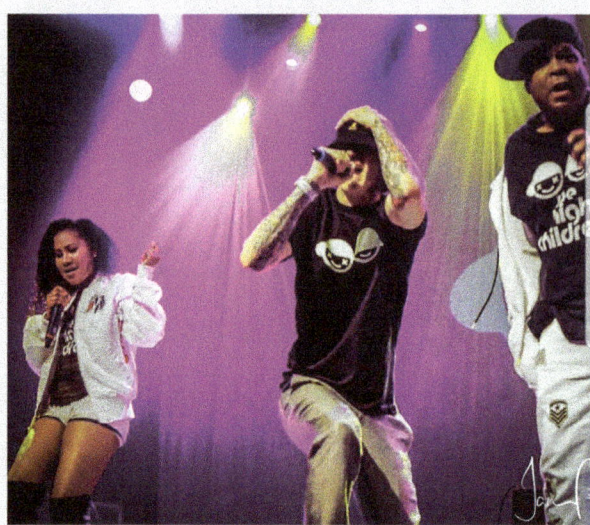
Jayson Ramos, Jamal Allen

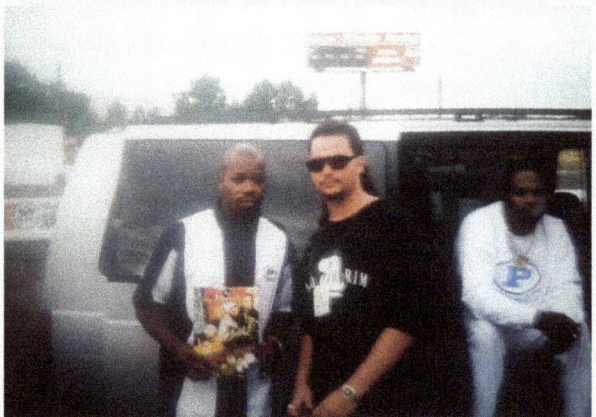
GrandMixer GMS & Too Short

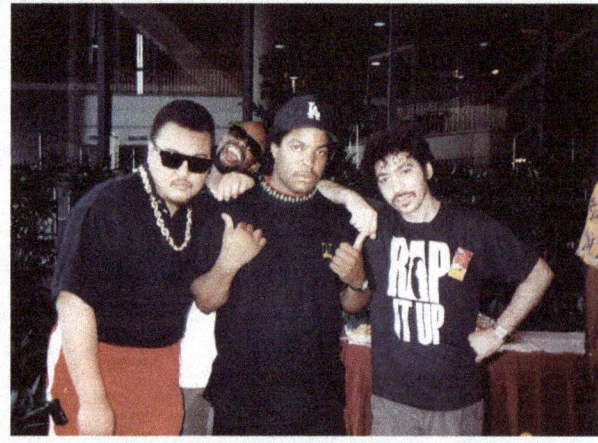
Nasty Nes, Ice Cube, Glen Ford

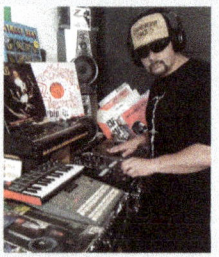
GrandMixer GMS

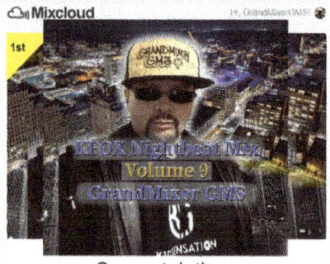
Congratulations

INTERVIEW WITH THE HIGH CHILDREN

Jayson Ramos, Jamal Allen, Nasty-Nes, Robbie Rob,
JJ Hudson aka Jmojii, Peter Morada, DJ 3rd Degree, GrandMixer GMS

1. GREAT TO HAVE YOU ON PUMP IT UP MAGAZINE. PLEASE, INTRODUCE YOURSELF?

We are The High Children, an open source Seattle-based hip hop band made up of Jayson Ramos, Jamal Allen, Nasty-Nes, Robbie Rob, JJ Hudson aka Jmojii, Peter Morada, DJ 3rd Degree, and the newest addition is GrandMixer GMS.

2. HOW DID YOU GET STARTED IN THE MUSIC BUSINESS?

Jmojii has been performing since the age of 4. She started with her love for all genres of dance including classical piano and invented her own style of 88 key runs. Nes started in radio at 18 on Seattle's 1250 KFOX and debuted the West Coast's first all rap radio show called "Freshtrack" in 1980. 3rd Degree began deejaying at 12 and did parties, dances, etc.; at 18 he worked at Tower Records which got his foot in the door. GMS began as a breakdancer at 11, he's self-taught, and began mixing on the radio in Spokane at 14. The High Children formed in the early 2000's, originally with Jayson, and then gradually expanded to include Jamal, Robbie Rob, Peter, and everyone else as time went by.

3. TELL US WHAT'S THE STORY BEHIND IT!

JJ is a domestic violence survivor and was modeling at a runway show. The High Children were to perform while she walked the catwalk. Right before the guests showed up, she noticed a grand piano. Whenever there is a piano she HAS to play! Jamal saw her, they talked, she began modeling for THC and going to the studio to learn and eventually recorded her first solo track, "Banger Banger." Nes introduced Seattle to Hip Hop music in 1980 and in 1983, to Sir Mix-A-Lot! 3rd Degree grew up as a DJ and breakdancer, was a buyer at Tower Records, did college radio and was in a few bands. He connected with many people over the years until meeting Nes, who was the biggest positive music connection. GMS taught himself how to mix to help his breakdancing battles for him and his cousin, Tony. When breakdancing died out in Spokane in the 80's, GMS transitioned to DJ'ing as a way to stay in Hip-Hop.

4. WHAT MAKES YOUR PRODUCTIONS UNIQUE? AND HOW WOULD YOU DESCRIBE IT? (GENRES/SUB-GENRES)?

JJ is a little old school with a new style and a unique tone to her rap style. Nes & GMS's mixing style is unique – not your basic mixing one song into another song but several songs using different beats and vocal effects similar to a remix and a lot like a mash up, something they were doing back in the 80's. GMS has stayed up-to-date with his scratching, but he doesn't overdo it and he mixes music from any genre. 3rd Degree also mixes different genres and his uniqueness comes from his ability to sing, rap and dance, and his rhyme-style has an updated old-school feel.
The group overall has a unique melodic singing/rap style with catchy hooks, and a fusion of multiple genres, from old school Hip-Hop, to EDM, R&B, Rock, Pop, and anything else that can be found. Our live, on-stage rap performances feature actual playing of Akai MPC's, EMU SP1200's, and using turntables as instruments.

THE HIGH CHILDREN

5. WHO ARE YOUR BIGGEST MUSICAL INFLUENCES? AND ANY PARTICULAR ARTIST/BAND YOU WOULD LIKE TO COLLABORATE WITH IN THE FUTURE?

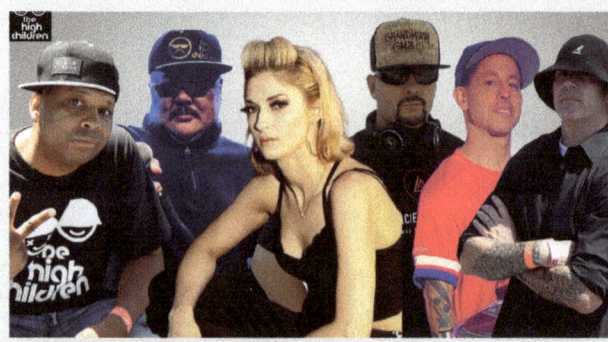

JJ grew up listening to a lot of 90's music. Her biggest influences: 2Pac, Biggy, Jay-Z, TLC, Drake. Locally, she would like to collaborate with Jordy Sams from Seattle or Cordell Drake from Spokane.

Nes' influences are The Osmond Brothers, David Cassidy, Spinners, Stylistics, Carpenters, Beatles, Sir Mix-A-Lot and NWA, and in life, Bruce Lee. 3rd Degree's influences are Run DMC, Eric B & Rakim, KRS One and BDP, A Tribe Called Quest, Public Enemy, Rage Against The Machine, Linkin Park, Marvin Gaye, and Duran Duran and would like to work with 9th Wonder and Masta Ace. GMS's influences are Nasty-Nes, the late Cameron Paul, the KDAY Mixmasters, The Latin Rascals, Alex Mejia, Prince Ice, Bob Rosenberg and every song that he grew up listening to. Robbie Rob is from Minneapolis and was influenced by a lot of the greats from there: Prince, Jimmy Jam & Terry Lewis and the Time, and many others

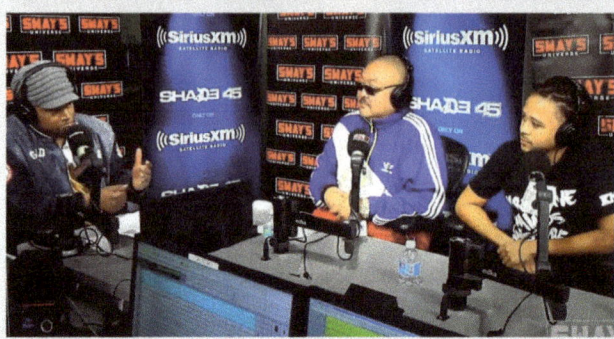

6. WHICH IS THE BEST MOMENT IN YOUR MUSICAL CAREER THAT YOU'RE MOST PROUD OF? (AWARDS, PROJECTS OR PUBLIC PERFORMANCES ETC)

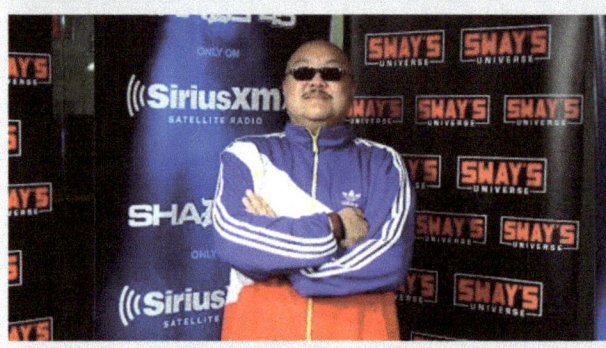

JJ has only been in the music business for three years Her favorite part is performing and seeing her fans in the crowd vibing out with her to her songs!

Nes' awards are the gold and platinum plaques from Michael Jackson, Whitney Houston, Sir Mix-A-Lot, De La Soul, Lauryn Hill, Chic, NWA & Eazy E, to name a few. 3rd Degree's best moments are his appearance on the "Sway In The Morning" show along with Nasty Nes, The High Children, and Kritta. Second would be his time in Super Dank Brothers performing at the iconic venues on the Sunset Strip in Hollywood, CA. For GMS, it's being the first DJ in Spokane to mix for commercial radio with TJ Collins on Power 104 and being the first Spokane DJ to showcase his turntable skills on "Sway In The Morning"; winning the 1993 Inland Northwest Battle of The DJ's; working with his influence, Nasty-Nes; his mixes and syndicated radio mixshow, "Global Frequency," going #1 on multiple Global Mixcloud charts; and working with West Coast pioneer, Tairrie B. Of course, we are all proud of JJ's song, "J," going #1 on RapAttackLives College Rap Radio Chart, and The High Children's song, "Masarap," going #1 on The Urban Influencer & Radio Airplay Experts' TOP 30 RAP RADIO CHART!

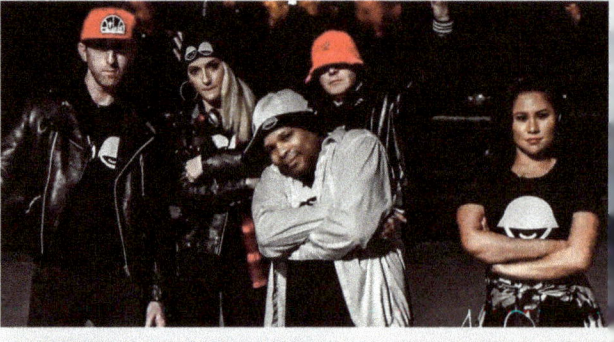

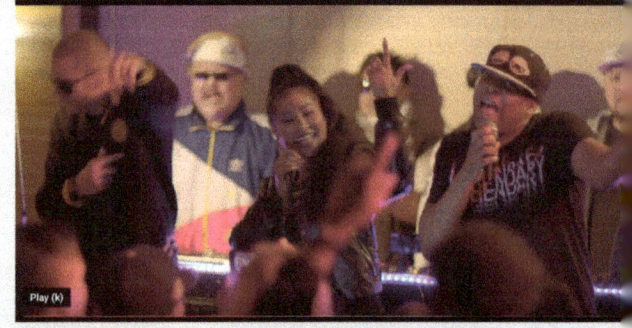

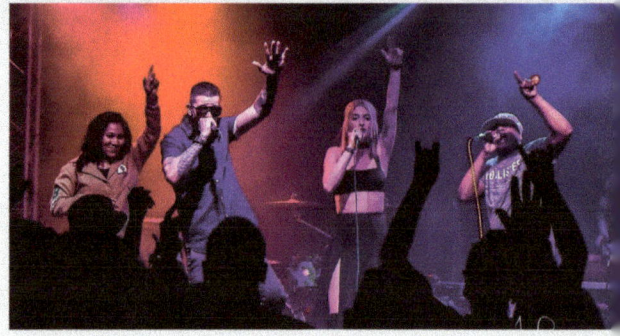

THE HIGH CHILDREN

7. WHAT ADVICE WOULD YOU GIVE TO ASPIRING DJS, MUSICIANS?

Have confidence, stay consistent, patient, focused, humble. Find a mentor in your field. Intern. Live, eat, and breathe your craft and work hard for your goals – even for free in the beginning. Develop a good network of like-minded people, don't be afraid to ask for help, ideas, feedback, and be willing to do the same. Treat everyone with respect, whether it's a secretary, intern, janitor, whoever, because everyone starts somewhere – even P. Diddy was an intern – and they will always remember if you were rude to them or their friend, who may have been the janitor. Tune out the negativity – only using it for motivation – and focus on moving forward, one step at a time. Set goals, write them down and follow through! Remember, it is a marathon, not a sprint!

8. WHAT'S NEXT FOR YOU? ANY UPCOMING PROJECTS OR TOURS?

Nes is going to become the biggest Filipino TV or movie star in the United States!

3rd Degree has a lot of new music to drop this year and is going on tour in the next year or so.
GMS is expanding his "Global Frequency" radio mixshow network; he's working on new music and remixes with Tairrie B, JJ Hudson, THC, 3rd Degree, Mak Music; and is booking tour dates, starting with Minneapolis in August and Brazil is on the horizon.
THC has a lot of new music coming up, including a collaboration with various artists about George Floyd.
JJ is going to keep grinding, creating new projects for her fans! She's releasing a new single this month called "Let it Pop," produced by her super producer Robbie Rob: it has an old school-yet-new-style vibe and is being released in perfect time to let it pop for your summer pool parties!

9. IF YOU HAD ONE MESSAGE TO GIVE TO YOUR FANS, WHAT WOULD IT BE?

JJ: "live in the moment because tomorrow is not promised and just enjoy life!" Nes: "don't do drugs or smoke cigarettes." 3rd Degree: "Thank you so very much for the love and support. I make music in hopes it will help move someone to a positive place." GMS: "Appreciate the little things and make the most of each moment in life because we only live once, do what makes you happy and each day strive to be a better version of yourself than you were yesterday!"

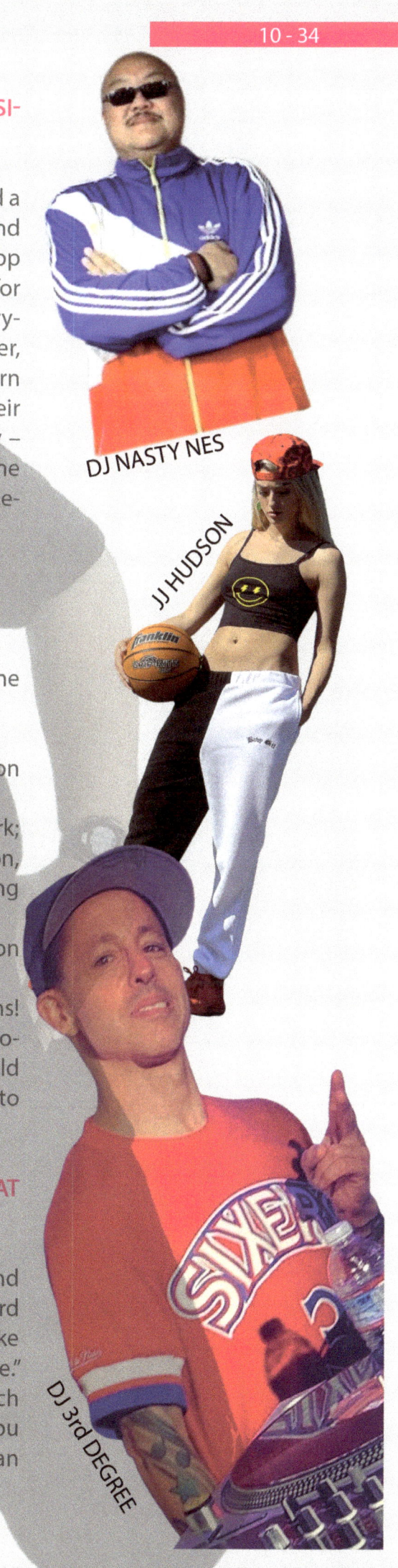

DJ NASTY NES
JJ HUDSON
DJ 3rd DEGREE

REVIEW

Make Music With The Power Of Your Mind With Next Mind - Oculus Quest 2

WHAT YOU THINK IS WHAT YOU DO

The image you see is projected onto your visual cortex

What you focus on is identified byu the sensor in real time

Use your focus to control your digital envronment

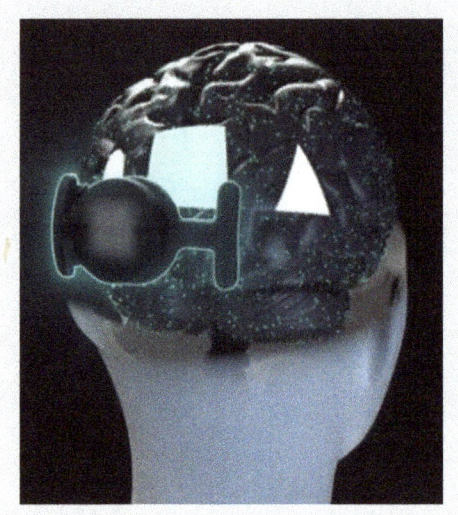

SMALL BUT POWERFUL

A compact, comb-shaped sensor offers comfort, discretion, and the best measurement of neural activity on the market.

NextMind Sensor. A brain-sensing wearable with an adjustable headband.

NextMind Engine. Real-time algorithms transform neural signals into commands.

GET INSTANT CONTROL

Once you're linked in, using your mind to control your digital environment is surprisingly easy.

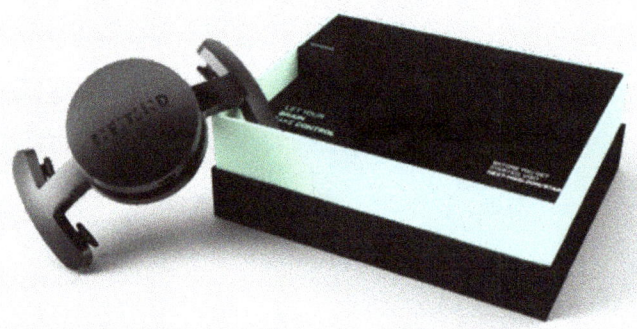

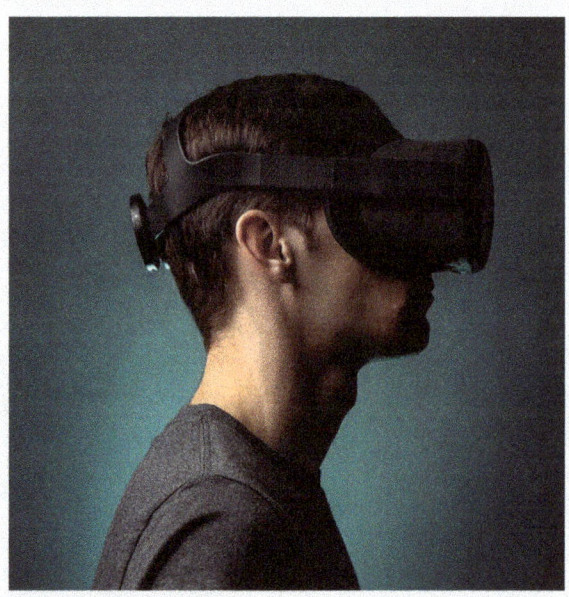

Pump it up Magazine / 11 - 32

CONTROLLING VIRTUAL REALITY WITH YOUR MIND

Let's face it. In the future, we won't be holding controllers to navigate in virtual reality experiences. Our brains will be sending commands and instructions directly to the device. But it's not the future. This post from Scott Stein at CNet shows how the technology is already available in a development prototype from the company NextMind. Any kind of widespread usage is most likely many years away but it's amazing to think how technology can read what we, well, think. It not only sounds fascinating but also intimidating and maybe even frightening. Just how much of our thoughts will technology be able to "read" and where will that data be kept? This takes the personal security argument to new levels as now our grey matter is being probed. Be careful what you think!

In my Oculus Quest VR headset, I was in a room surrounded by large-brained aliens. Their heads flashed, white and black. I turned to one, staring at it. Soon enough, its head exploded. I looked at the others, making their heads explode. Then I looked at a flashing portal marker across the room and was gone. I did this without eye tracking. A band on the back of my head was sensing my visual cortex with electrodes.

I felt like I was living some sort of real-life virtual version of the David Cronenberg film, Scanners. But in reality, I was trying a neural input device made by NextMind.

Before holiday break, I received a large black box with a small package inside. A black disc, with a headband. The disc was covered in small rubber-footed pads. NextMind's $399 developer kit, announced a year ago at CES 2020, aims at something many companies are striving for: neural inputs. NextMind aims to read a brain's signals to track attention, control objects and maybe even more.

It's hard to understand the real potential and possibilities of neural input technology. Also, many of the startups in this space are doing different things. CTRL-Labs, a neurotechnology company acquired by Facebook in 2019, developed an armband that could send hand and finger inputs. Another company, Mudra, is making a wristband for Apple Watch later this year that also senses neural inputs on the wrist.

I wore an early version of the Mudra Band a year ago, and experienced how it could interpret my finger's movements, and even roughly measure how much pressure I was applying when I squeezed my fingers. Even more weirdly, Mudra's tech can work when you aren't moving your fingers at all. The applications could include assisting people who don't even have hands, like a prosthetic wearable.

NextMind's ambitions look to follow a similar assistive-tech path, while also aiming for a world where neural devices could possibly help improve accuracy with physical inputs — or combine with a world of other peripherals. Facebook's AR/VR head, Andrew Bosworth, sees neural input tech emerging at Facebook within three to five years, where it could end up being combined with wearable devices like smart glasses.

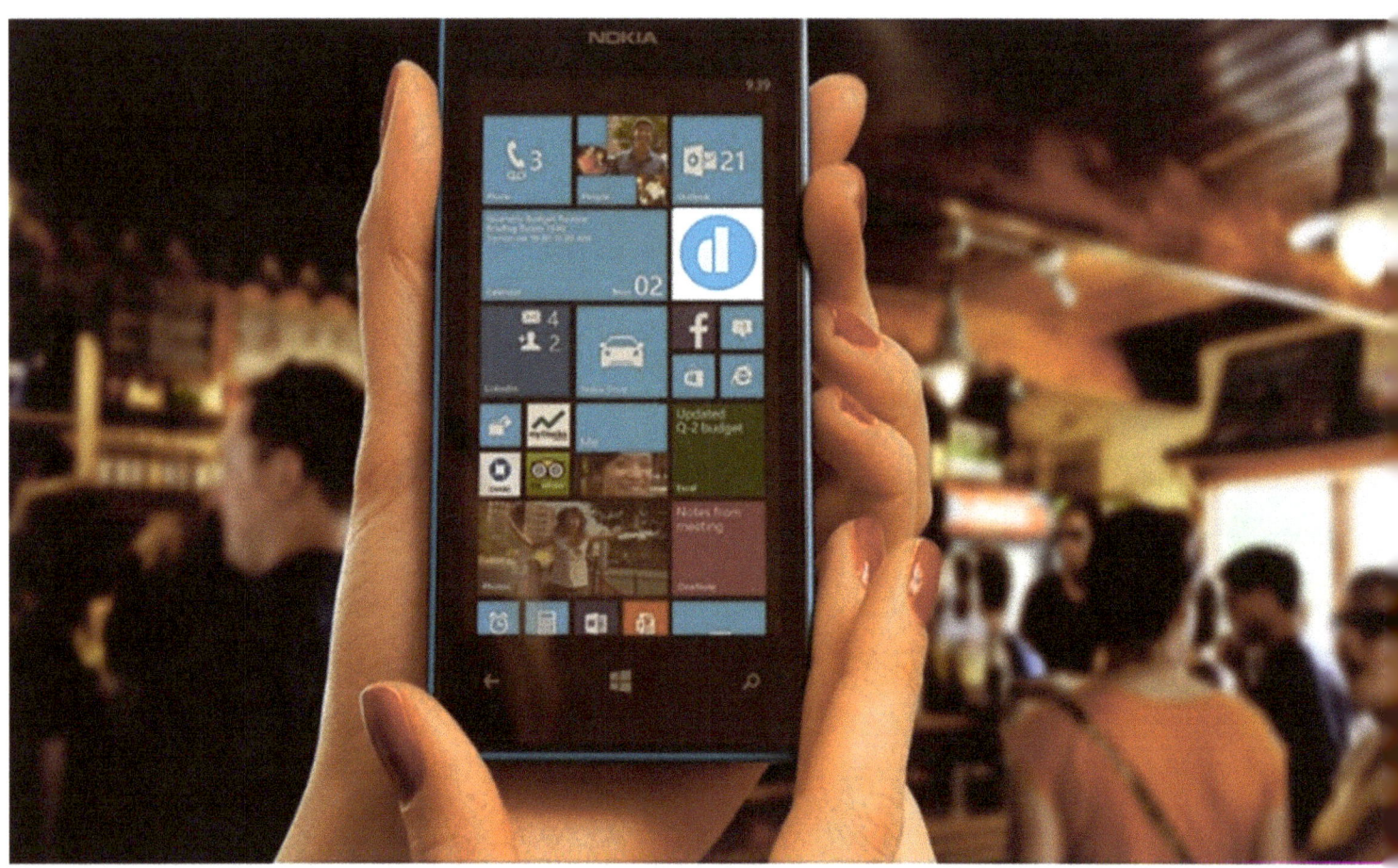

FESTIVALS

GET READY TO DANCE
BEST MUSIC FESTIVALS 2021

Floydfest 2021
When: July 21-25, 2021

Where: Floyd, VA

The Scene: The homegrown Floydfest has only one modest aim: "Our mission is to the be the best music experience of our time." The lofty promise is generating results as each year the lineup gets deeper and the names get bigger. The famous Blue Ridge Parkway serves as your living room for the weekend.

The Lineup: Keller Williams, Leftover Salmon, Old Crow Medicine Show, The Avett Brothers

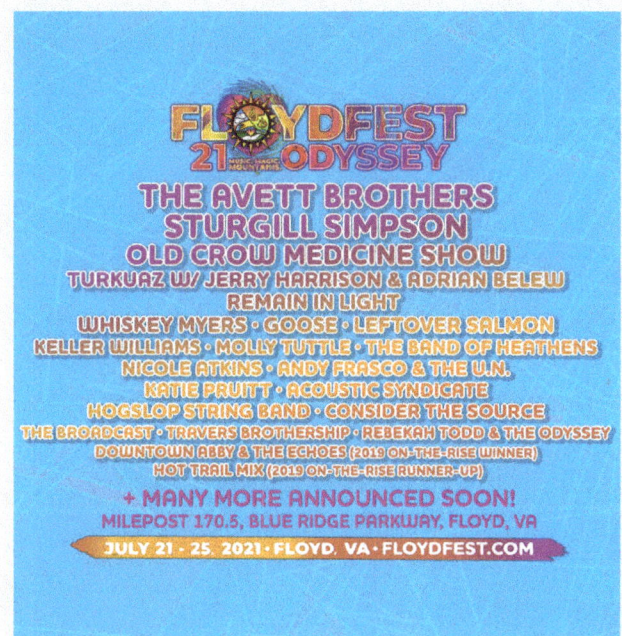

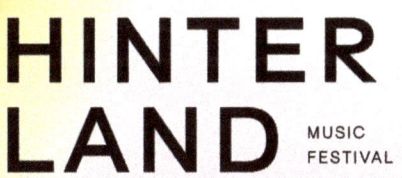

Hinterland Festival 2021
When: August 6-8, 2021

Where: Des Moines, IA

The Scene: Strike out for the uncharted regions of central Iowa and the two-day Hinterland Festival. Located along the scenic Raccoon River, this newcomer to the festival scene has already hosted a number of world class bands including San Fermin, TV on the Radio, Future Islands, Shakey Graves, Dwight Yoakam, and Ryan Adams.

The Lineup: Old Crow Medicine Show, The Avett Brothers

GET READY TO DANCE
BEST MUSIC FESTIVALS 2021

Summer Camp 2021
When: August 20-22, 2021

Where: Chillicothe, IL

The Scene: From chilled out late night campfire jams to beat busting dance shows, the party at Summer Camp goes long past the end of scheduled performances. 'Scampers' can apply to become camp counselors which means free tickets, free camping, and free beer in exchange for being an official party ambassador to the other attendees. Our resident festival expert calls Summer Camp — 'The best festival of the Memorial Day Weekend.

The Lineup: EOTO, Griz, Keller Williams, Lettuce, Rezz, Shpongle, The Werks, Umphrey's McGee, Ween

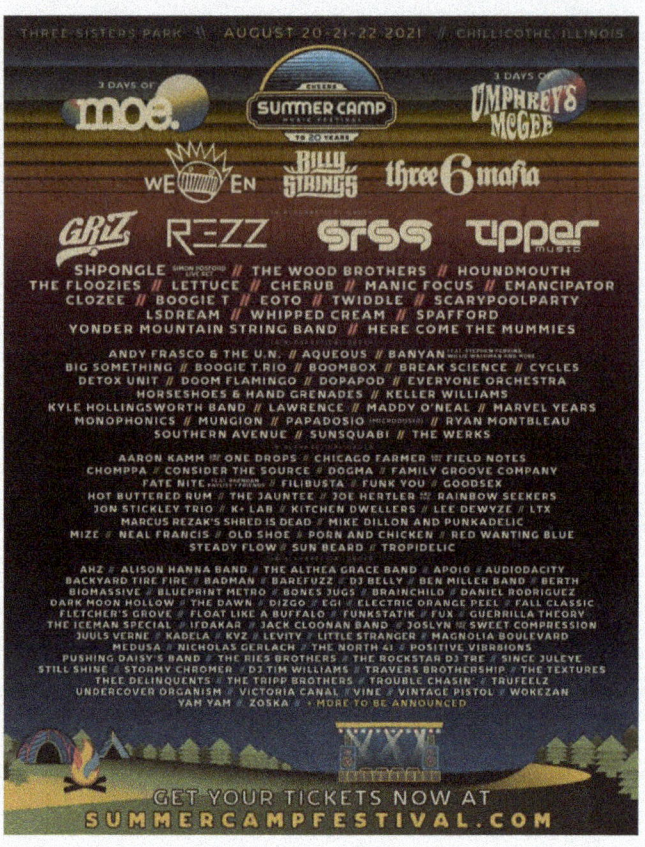

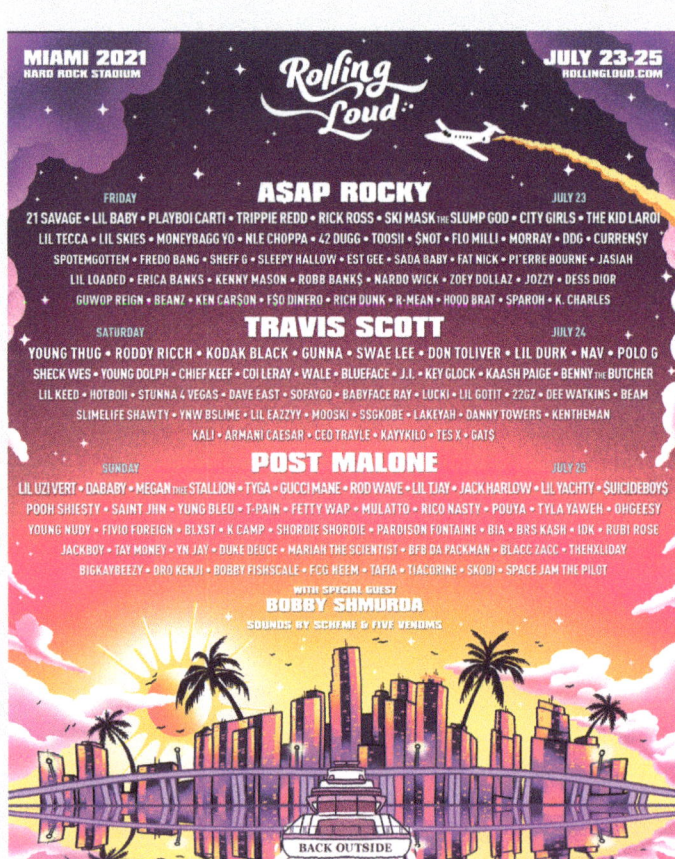

Rolling Loud Miami 2021
When: July 23-25, 2021

Where: Miami, FL

The Scene: The largest hip-hop festival in the world is a three-day event that started in Miami, Florida. Some of the biggest names in the business have already played this newcomer to the Florida festival scene including Kendrick Lamar, Future, Lil Wayne, A$AP Rocky, Travis Scott, Young Thug, Lil B, Post Malone, Migos, Kodak Black, Lil Uzi Vert, 21 Savage, Lil Yachty, and more.

The Lineup: A$AP Rocky, Post Malone, Travis Scott

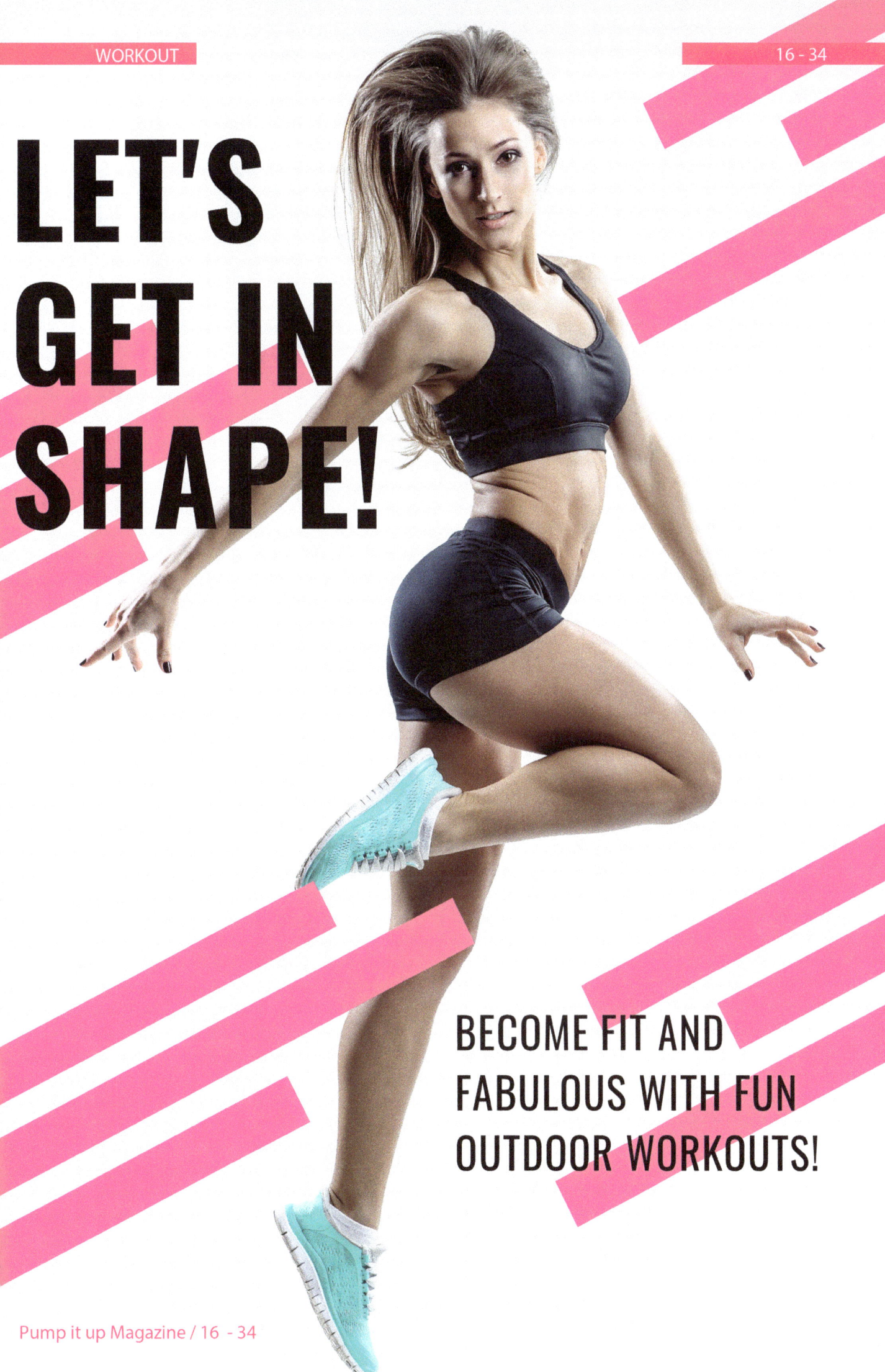

DITCH THE GYM AND TRY THESE OUTDOOR ACTIVITIES

Soak up the sun (just don't forget the SPF!)
with these great outdoor exercises that make outdoor workouts seem like playtime.

WALKING

Why get stuck on the treadmill when the weather is so beautiful? Walking is a great way to get outdoors, breathe in some fresh air and sneak in your daily workout. Walking at a moderate pace can burn 280 calories an hour in a 150-pound adult.

Getting yourself a fitness tracker could help. A small 2015 study found that nearly three of four participants maintained or increased their step goals by week 4 of a 16-week program while wearing a tracker. No need to purchase a fancy tracker when you could use your phone. The Sharecare app (available on iOS and Android) has a step counter to help you track your progress and stay motivated.

SWIMMING AND WATER EXERCISE

When it's hot outside, it feels great to take a dip in the pool, ocean or lake. According to the Centers for Disease Control and Prevention (CDC), swimming and other water-based exercises offer a number of benefits, especially for people with arthritis. Swimming helps those with rheumatoid arthritis more than other fitness activities. Water-based exercise also improves joint health and decreases pain in people with osteoarthritis. You don't even need to do laps—just swimming leisurely can burn more than 400 calories an hour

BIKING

Riding a bike is a fun way to get where you're going—and get fit on your way there. An easy ride can burn 290 calories an hour, while more vigorous pedaling can burn nearly 600. Unfortunately, there are several injuries associated with biking. Hospital admissions for bike injuries more than doubled from 1999 to 2013, so make sure to wear a helmet and bright, reflective clothing, and follow the rules of the road.

GARDENING AND YARD WORK

Staying fit might be a compelling reason to knock out some of your chores. Light gardening or pushing a lawnmower can burn about 330 calories per hour. Cut the grass, plant some flowers and two hours later you'll have burned the equivalent of a Big Mac, with a little room to spare.

LAWN SPORTS

Now that you've mowed the lawn, it's time to play yard games. Playing a game of Frisbee or horseshoes will burn about 200 calories an hour, and croquet can burn 225. But if you really want to turn up the heat, try Ultimate Frisbee. It's fun, fast-paced and can help you shed 544 calories.

Enjoy The Sound Of
Pump it up
RADIO

Get the free Pump it up magazine Radio App on your smartphone or tablet, and you'll never miss your favourite music!

POP - ROCK - DANCE - RNB - JAZZ
Available on Google Play Store

www.PumpItUpMagazine.com

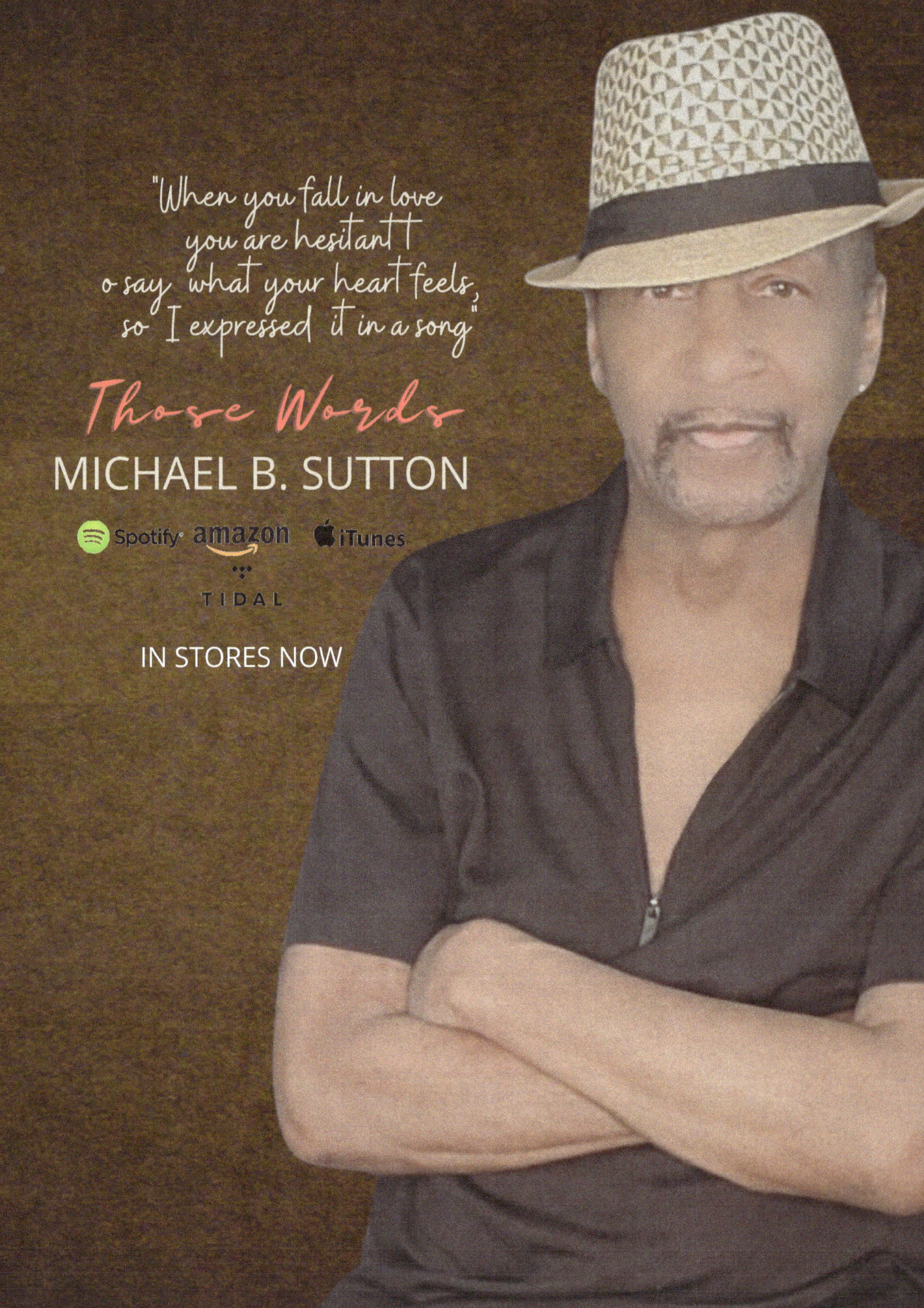

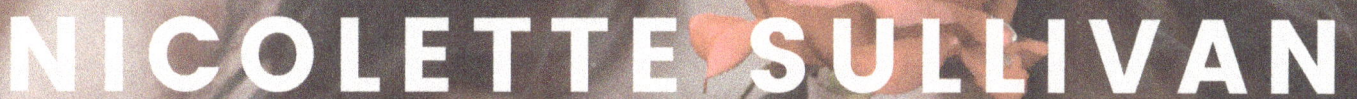

NICOLETTE SULLIVAN

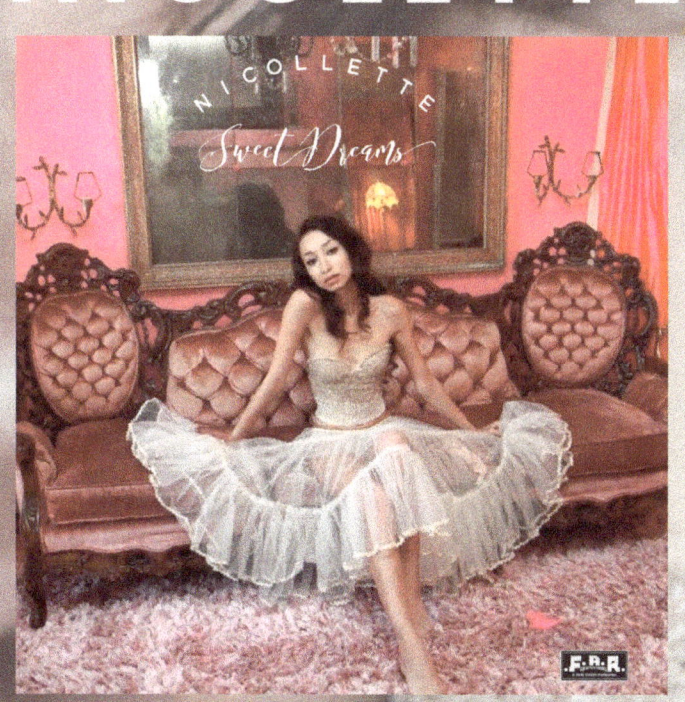
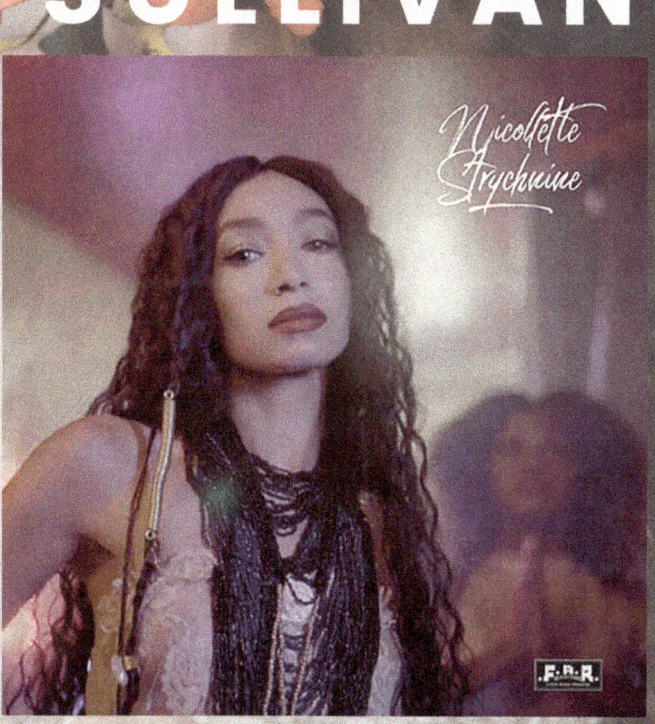

Spotify amazon iTunes
TIDAL

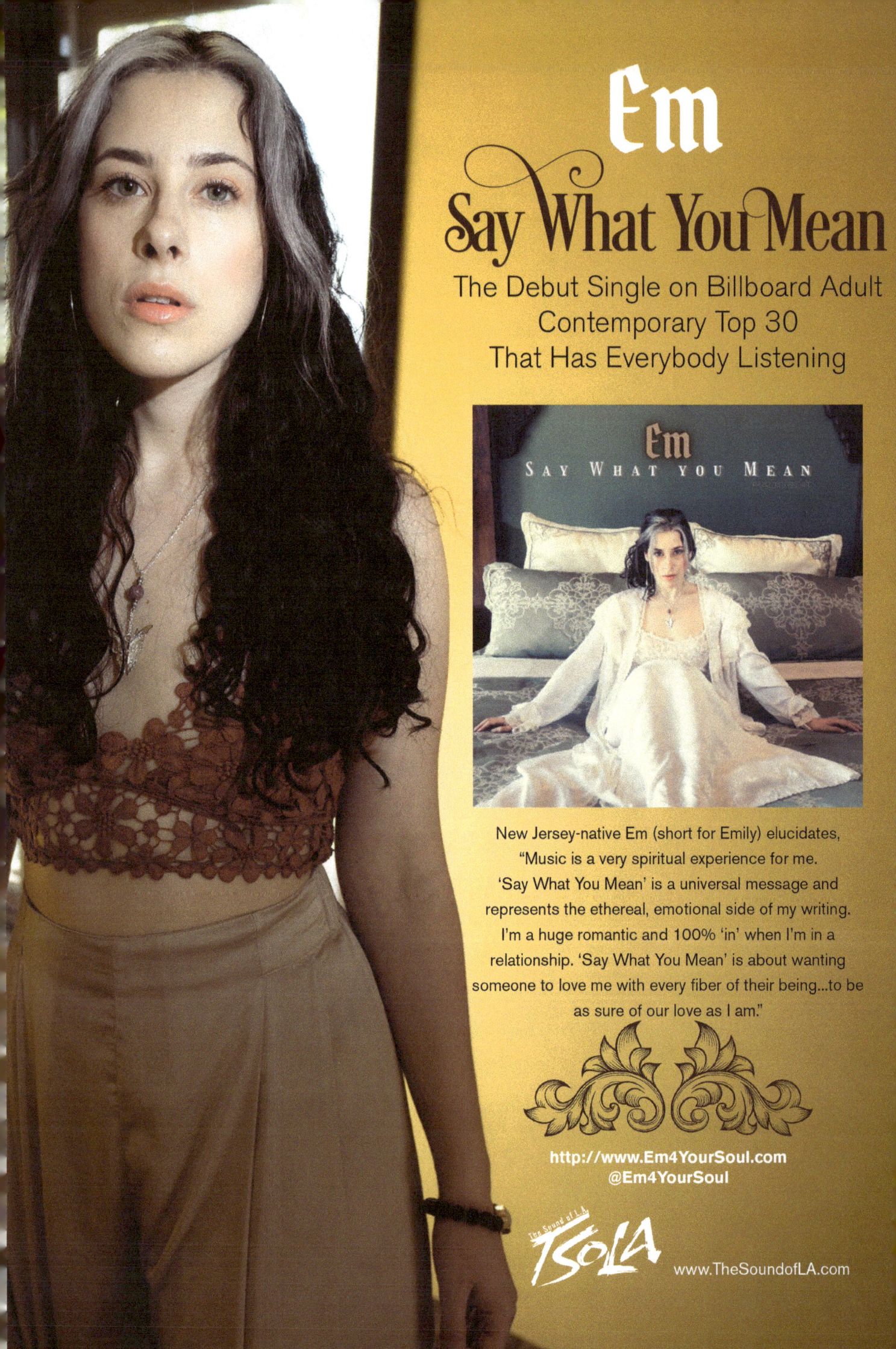

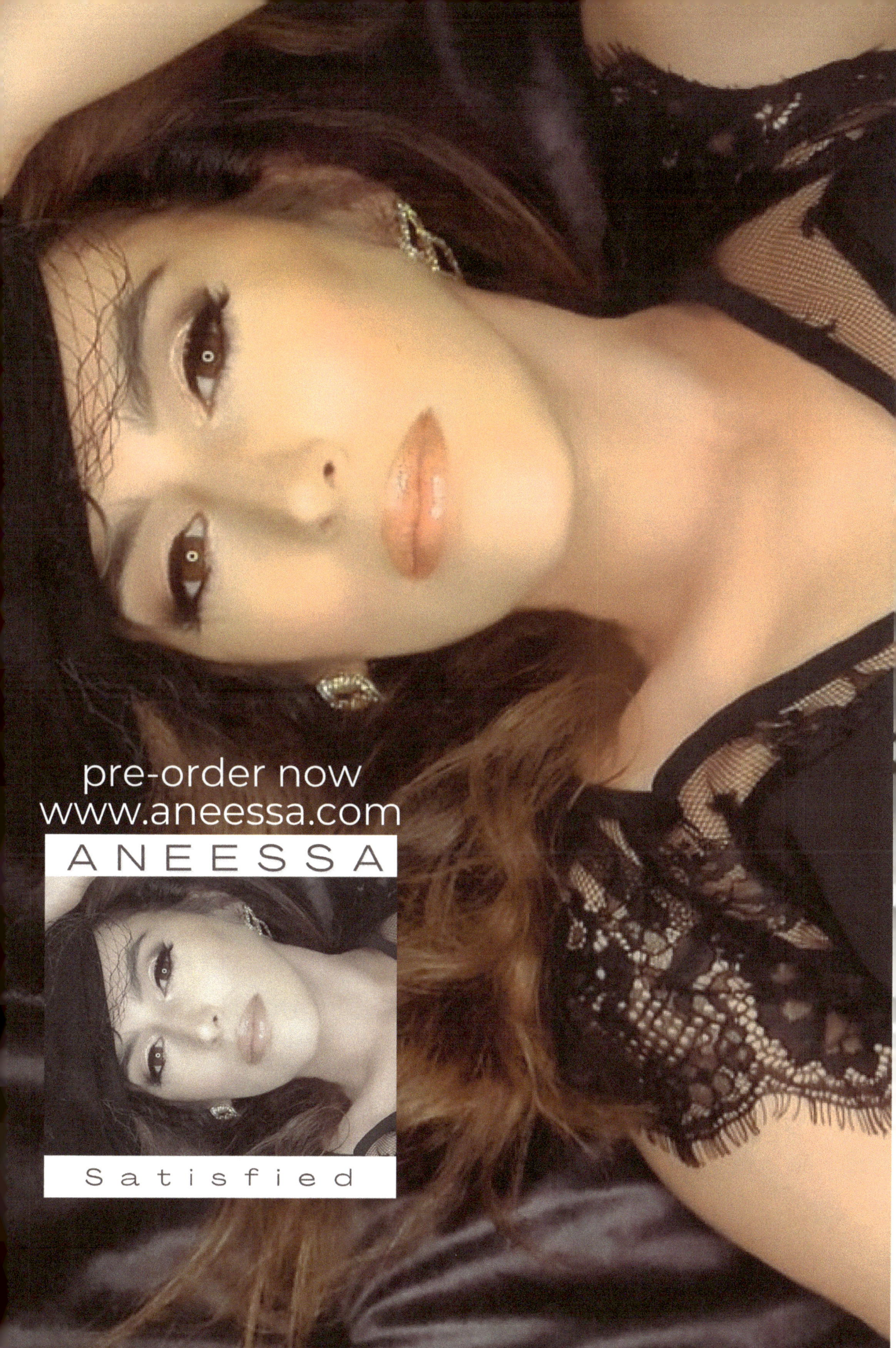

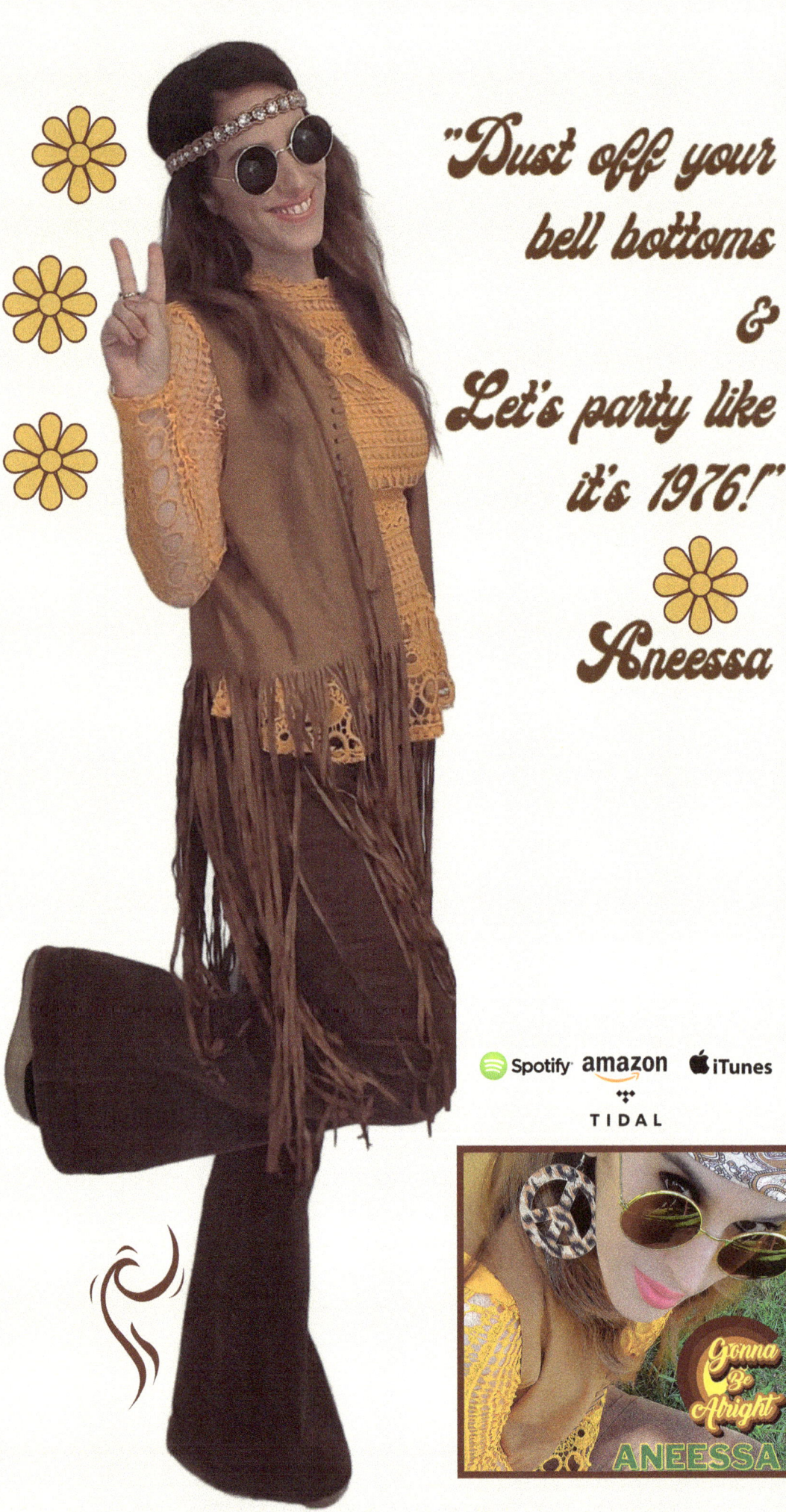

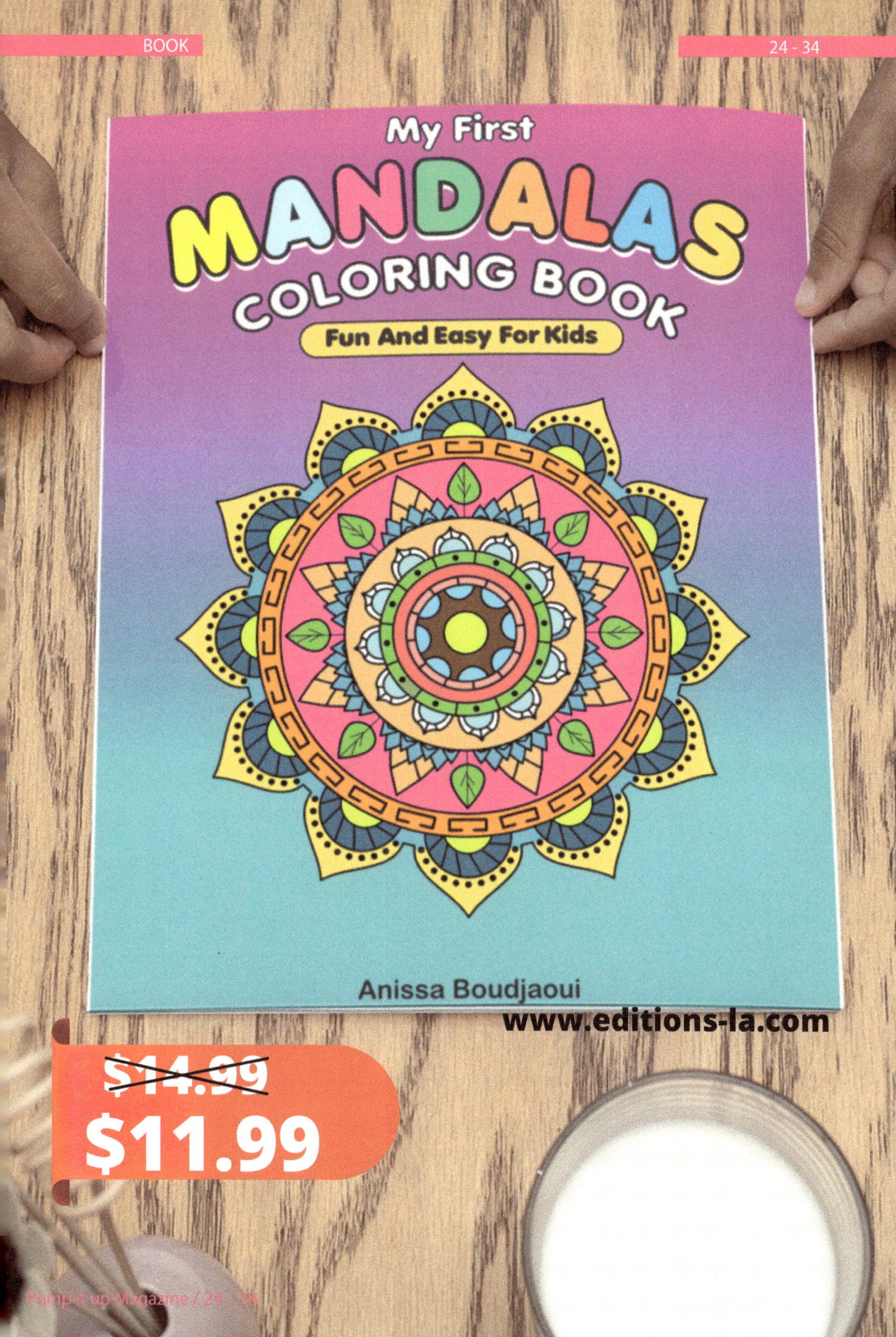

Paulette C. Jackson, Published Author and Acclaimed Radio Personality, Releases Latest Book "MyTest(Imony)"

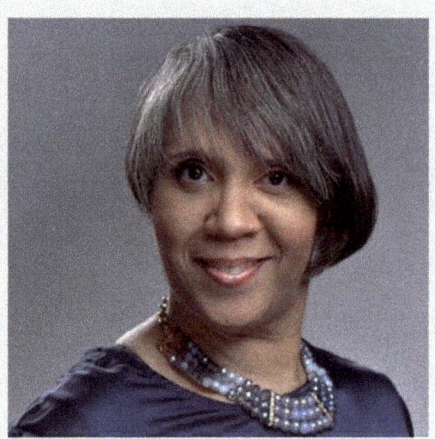

The author's latest publication comes after back-to-back successes from her previous books, both of which were recently accepted for consideration for the 2020 Author Academy Awards. Paulette C. Jackson, Founder/CEO of SCORP Radio Network and Jazz Zone Radio, has released her latest book, "My Test(Imony)" on January 11, 2021. The book is the third publication by the published author, whose previous books "The Music in Me" and "The Music Through the Storm" both were recently accepted for consideration for the 2020 Author Academy Awards

Speaking about the book, Paulette stated during a recent interview, "I never really focused on writing books until the later part of my career, but I always knew I had it in me to be an author someday. My Test(Imony) is the third book I've released thus far, and it goes to show you that anything is possible and unexpected blessings are indeed, very real!"

Paulette is also renowned as the host of "The Classic Soul Music Café," "The Jazz Zone," and "Center Stage" Internet Radio Shows while simultaneously running her own business Ms. Music's Voice, as Voiceover Artist. The acclaimed radio personality began working with several artists on promotions and show bookings, and one of these ventures led to the creation of several video series and other creative projects, including SCORP Lady Ventures. She is also a part of ASCAP (American Society of Composers, Authors, and Publishers) as a songwriter and music publisher. Apart from these accomplishments, Paulette was also recently selected to receive the 2nd Annual Aretha Franklin Lifetime Achievement Award. The first to receive this honor was none other than Mary Wilson of the world-famous Supremes. Paulette will be receiving her honor at the 2020 National Rhythm & Blues Induction Ceremony (10th year anniversary) in Detroit, MI, later this year in 2021.

According to Paulette, her love for music and entertainment has always occupied her and kept her working in different business areas throughout these years.

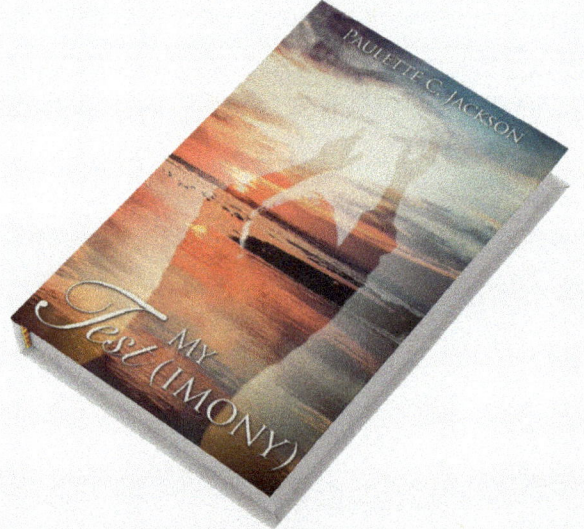

The author's latest book is available now on Amazon (paperback and eBook) and Barnes & Noble
Available on other book retailers
For more information, visit her official website now at time I launched two internet radio stations, SCORP Radio Network (Classic R&B, Soul) and Jazz Zone Radio (All types of Jazz).

Website: www.scorpladyventures.com

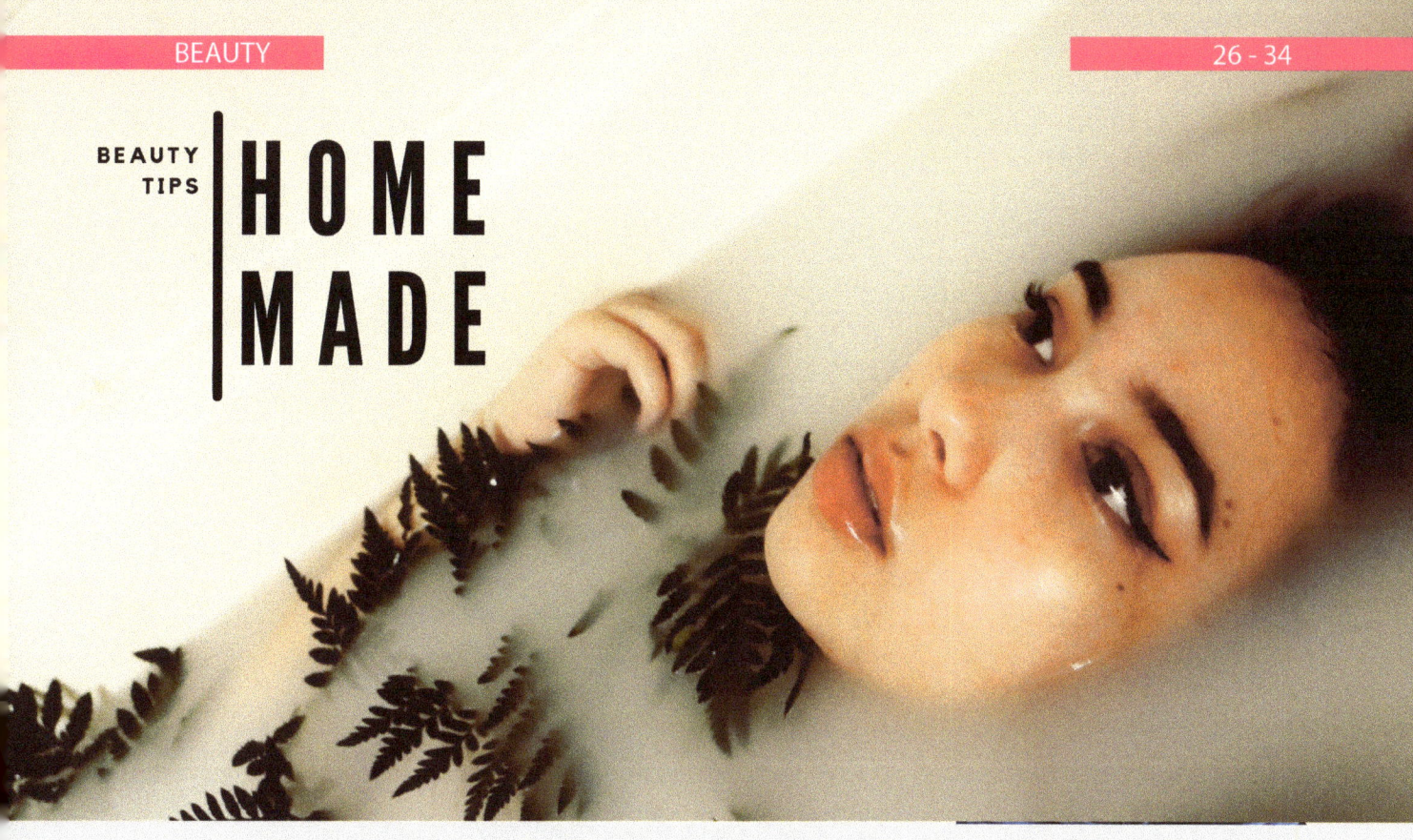

BEAUTY TIPS | HOME MADE

ESSENTIAL AND NATURAL FACELIFTING HOME REMEDIES TIPS THAT PEOPLE SHOULD DEFINITELY TRY OUT AND FOLLOW ON A REGULAR BASIS.

1. AVOCADO AND RICE POWDER MASK:

This is not only a mask but this is also an exfoliator. This is very good for people having dry and sagging surface. People who has dryness and needs Moisturization they can benefit with this. The powder will help to exfoliate and the avocado contains excellent moisturising properties. These can be very helpful.

People can mix about 1 cup of pulp of avocado which should be ripe and to this about half a teaspoon of grained rice powder.
This should be applied normally and then after 20 minutes, this should be washed off by scrubbing in gentle motions.
The mask will soften the surface and then it can be scrubbed easily.
This should be done as per requirement which can be twice a week.

2. LEMON JUICE AND OLIVE OIL MASSAGE FOR FAIRNESS SKIN:

This is very good for those having sagging and old surface. This can be good for those who have clogged pores because warm olive oil will help to open the ores. At the same time, the lemon juice helps to mildly bleach the surface and give a glowing effect.
About 1 teaspoon of good brand olive oil can be taken and slightly warmed up.
To this about 1 teaspoon of fresh lemon juice can be mixed.
Massage on for about 6 minutes and then wash off with a cleanser.
This should only be done a few times a week.
This should be avoided or the lemon juice used in less quantity if these is irritating to the person using this.

3. TEA BAG SOAK FOR TIRED EYES:

This is a very popular method to soothe the tired eyes. People having dry or dullness around the eyelids, can try soaking tea bags in warm water and then take these to get chilled in the refrigerator.
Then these can be put directly over the area and then the person can lie down for about 15 minutes. This is the treatment time. Then the eyes and also the surrounding area will feel freshen. This can regularly be followed to get rid of any patches or even bags.

4. EGG WHITE & HONEY MASK

Egg whites and honey have each been known for their many health benefits. But together, the two foods can also be combined and used as a mask to tighten sagging and loose skin.

Egg white is rich in the protein albumin, which works to rebuild skin cells, improve skin's elasticity, and impart a natural glow. Honey is a powerful antioxidant that can help remove toxins that build up over time in your skin. Used together, they provide a powerful one-two punch to tighten skin.

Separate 1 egg white from the yolk. Mix the egg white with 2 tablespoons of honey and apply it to your face, neck, or chest. Leave the mixture on for 15 minutes. After the 15 minutes, wash off the mask with warm water and pat dry. For best results, use the egg white and honey mask once a week.

5. 4. COFFEE SCRUB

offee is the go-to morning beverage for millions of people. Not only can coffee help you start your day, it can also be used at night to tighten your skin and prevent the signs of aging.
Coffee contains antioxidants that slow the signs of skin aging. When used as a scrub in combination with other substances, coffee exfoliates and firms your skin while at the same time working to smooth out and eliminate fat deposits.

In a bowl, combine the following ingredients:

¼ cup of coffee grounds
¼ cup of brown sugar
½ teaspoon of cinnamon
2 tablespoons of coconut oil (heat this slightly to make it a liquid)

6. BANANA

Bananas are a beauty powerhouse! They are rich in iron, zinc, potassium, magnesium, and vitamins A, B, C, and D. Mash a ripe banana and combine it with a few drops of fresh lemon juice Use the mixture as a mask and leave it on for 10 to 15 minutes before rinsing with warm water. Its minerals and vitamins pack the mask with anti-aging properties. Bonus: it also smooths and moisturizes your skin!

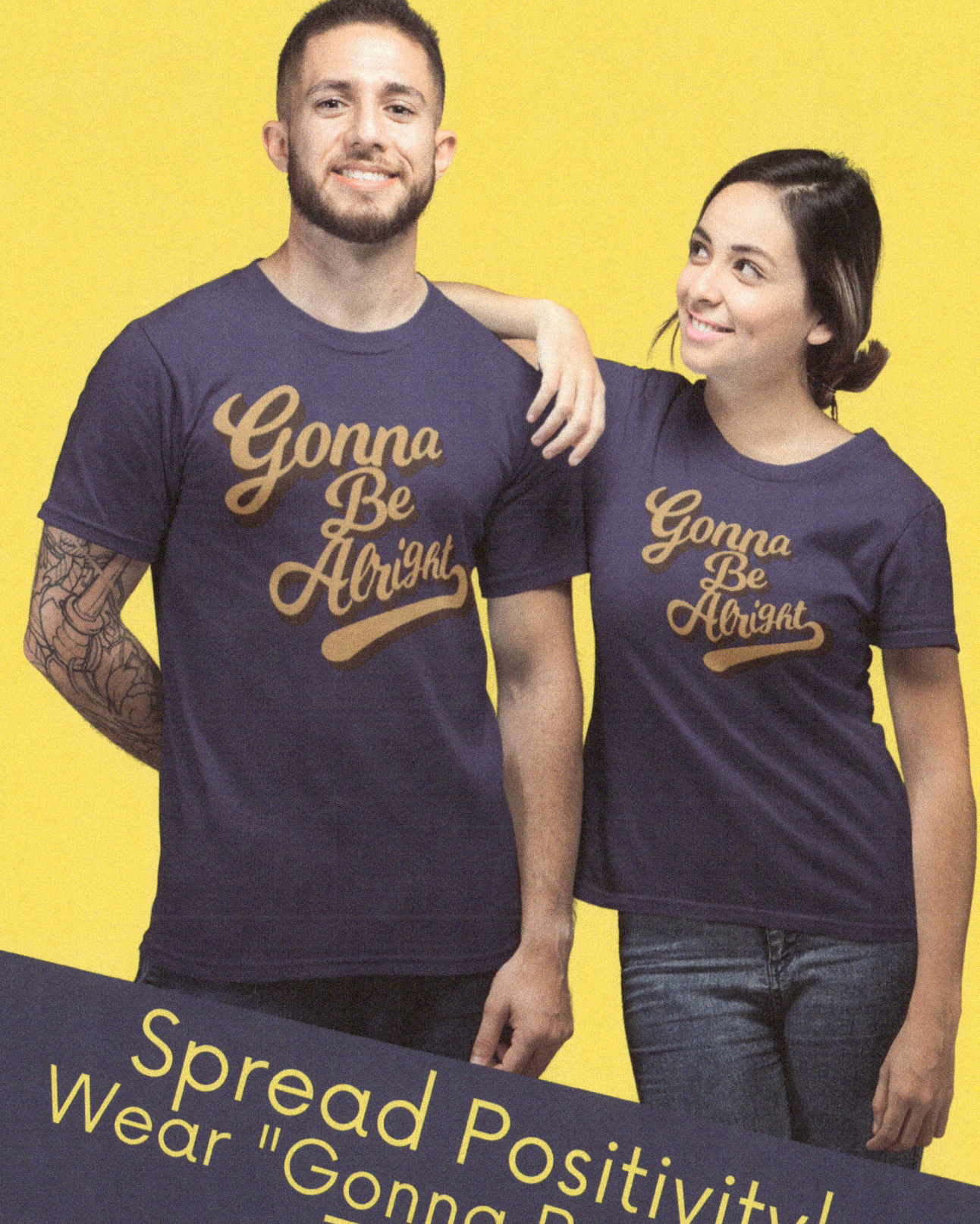

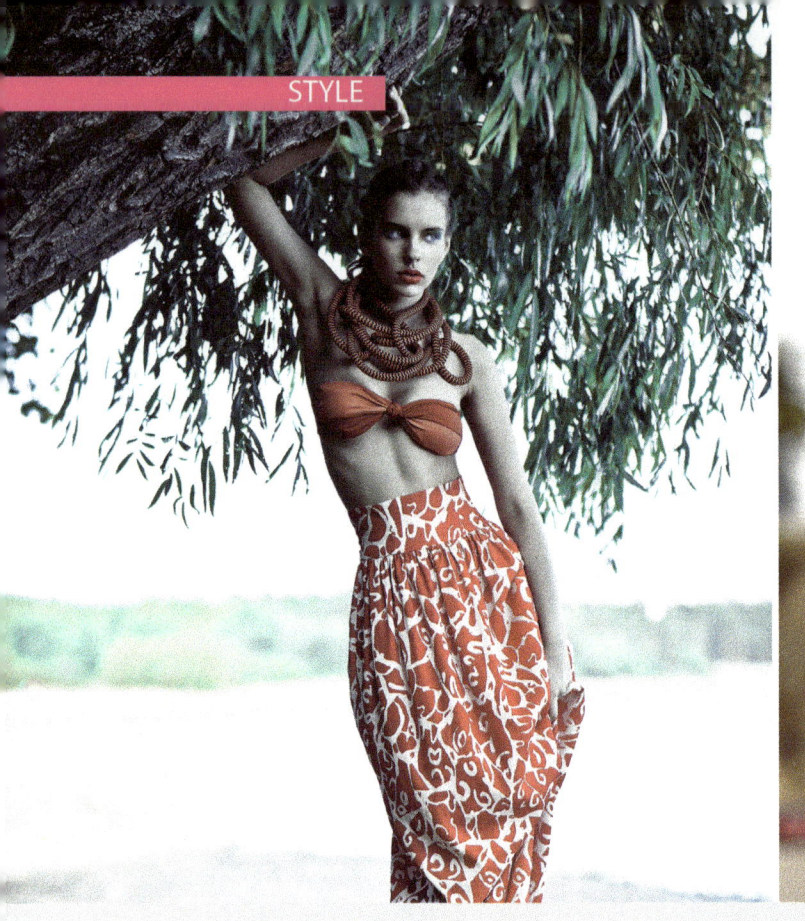
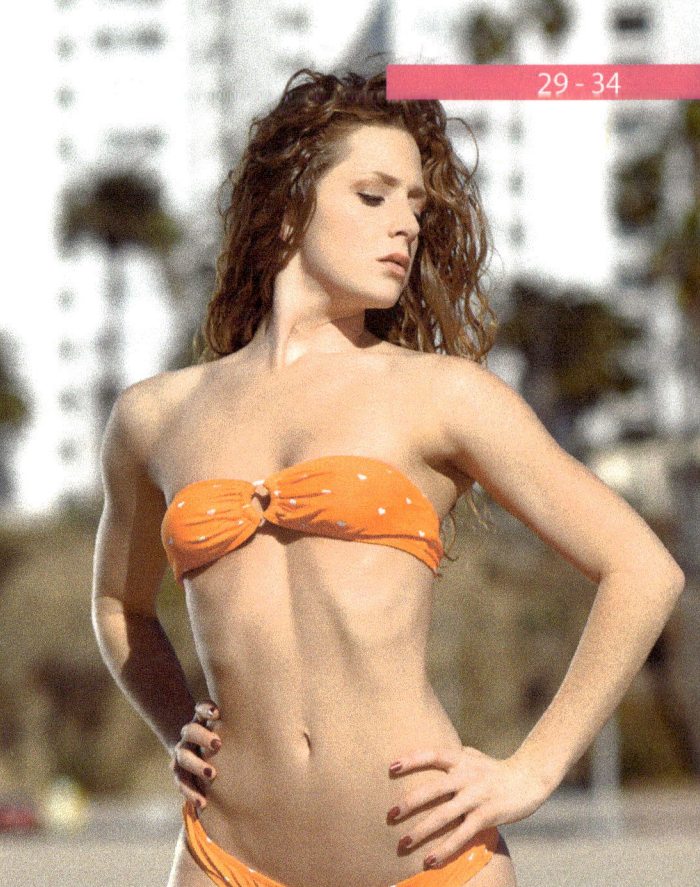

1. BANDEAU AND HIGH-WAISTED TROUSERS

Behold the effortlessly cool look of the summer: a bandeau bikini styled with a high-waisted, loose-fitting trouser. The best part? You can repeat this look hundreds of times with different colors, fabrics, and of course, accessories. Opt for a classic look with subtle hints of gold jewelry like a medium-sized hoop earring and dainty choker necklace.

2. BEACH KAFTAN OUTFIT

Just because beach dressing has evolved does not mean the classic kaftan cover-up is no longer in style—it just got the minimalist makeover. Pair the oversized kaftan with a strappy sandal—our go-to is The Row's Constance sandal— rectangular acetate sunglass, and chunky gold jewelry to complete the look.

3. BIKINI AND SILK BANDANA BEACH FASHION

Perhaps our favorite styling piece for the summer is the silk bandana. It's the ultimate versatile piece, from wearing it as a neck scarf or hair tie to a skirt or top; the silk bandana can be transformed into many different pieces. Our expert advice? Indulge in fun, bright prints and style with a basic black swimsuit.

4. STRIPED SWEATER AND HIGH-WAISTED DENIM SHORTS

This outfit will forever be a class beach look—especially when the weather errs on the cooler side. Update the striped sweater and denim cut-offs look by layering them over Jacquemus' strappy one-piece swimsuit and a sleek, leather tote bag.

HOW TO MAKE A LIVING WITH YOUR MUSIC

Do you need to "know somebody" or "get lucky" to build a fan base and grow an income as an artist?
Absolutely not!

BUILD AN EMAIL LIST.

Here's what I did… and what I recommend YOU do if you want to grow a fan base and grow an income. It's really a simple process. Grow an email list full of fans, and build a genuine relationship with them over time. Then invite them to buy your songs.

MAKE FRIENDS WITH YOUR NEW SUBSCRIBERS.

Be genuine. Be real. Be open. Be honest.
Give them an insider's look into your process. Tell them real stories about the real you. Don't disrespect them by hammering them with nonstop sales messages!
Give them things they'd never get if they weren't on your list. Make them look forward to hearing from you! If you do these things, they will buy your music — even today, when they don't have to buy ANY music from ANYONE. Your "secret ninja weapon" is a genuine connection with your fans.

ADVERTISING

In the heyday of pop and rock, musicians rarely wanted to be associated with corporate brands, but that's changing with the rise of rap as America's most popular genre. Brand partnerships offer artists the ability to sponsor or endorse a brand they might genuinely like, and get access to an additional revenue stream while they're at it. Another way musicians find side money is from YouTube monetization, wherein YouTube videos share in the profit from the ads that come tagged onto them. Psy's "Gangnam Style" reportedly made $2 million from 2 billion YouTube views. YouTube's head of music Lyor Cohen wrote in a blog post last year that YouTube's payout rate in the U.S. is as high as $3 per 1000 streams.

FASHION, MERCHANDISING, AND OTHER DIRECT SELLS

Selling non-music products like perfumes, paraphernalia and clothing lines is an easy money-making strategy that artists have been taking advantage of for decades — but in the digital era, musicians can also get creative with their methods, expanding well beyond traditional merch tents at concerts and posters on a website.

Artists are also starting to ask for money from audiences directly — via crowdfunding or creating custom channels of communication with their fans — outside of social media platforms like Instagram and Twitter. The Voice star Angie Johnson raised roughly $36,000 on Kickstarter to record an upcoming album, for instance. More groups are releasing dedicated apps or subscription packages for their music or selling bespoke products like artist-curated festivals, email subscriptions and limited music releases. Pitbull has his own cruise.

STREAMING

The music industry has now accepted streaming as its revenue-leader and is poised to adapt around that, with many analysts and experts expecting that the business will streamline itself — with rewrites of law, new royalties negotiations, mergers, acquisitions and consolidations — into something leaner and, finally, more lucrative for musicians. Bad news: No one knows when that will be.

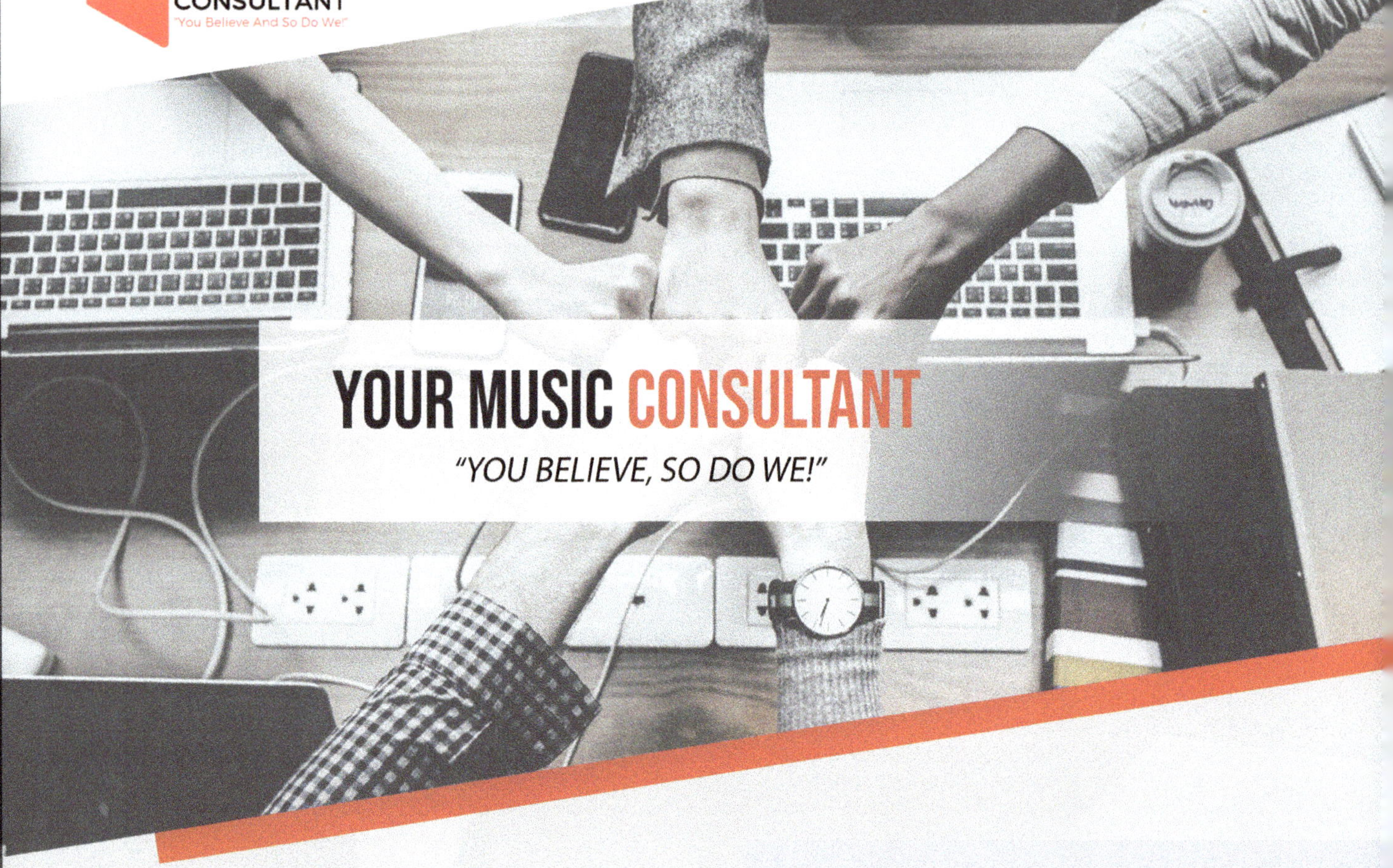

YOUR MUSIC CONSULTANT

"YOU BELIEVE, SO DO WE!"

We Can Help You To Grow Your Business

We are a monthly based service, we put faith in artists who has major potential, believed in them, and who are willing to spend their time and own money to work with us in building a successful music career!

Digital Marketing Services

SOCIAL MEDIA - STREAMING SERVICES - MUSIC DISTRIBUTION - PRESS RELEASE - PRESS DISTRIBUTION - PR

Radio Airplay and TV Commercial

TERRESTRIAL AND DIGITAL RADIO CAMPAIGN AL GENRES EXCEPT HEAVY METAL - CABLE TV AND MAJOR NETWORK COMMERCIAL

Licensing & Booking

CONCERTS, LIVE MUSIC, EVENTS, CLUB NIGHTS - RED CARPETS -
FOREIGN LICENSING AND SUBOPUBLISHING

Why Choose Us ?

3 DECADES OF MUSIC BUSINESS EXPERIENCE
Platinum and Gold Records

MOTOWN RECORDS
UNIVERSAL
SONY
CAPITOL RECORDS

WE WORKED WITH:
Kanye West - Jay Z - Stevie Wonder - Michael Jackson - Germaine Jackson Smokey Robinson - Dionne Warwick - Cheryl Lynn - The Originals -

📞 **1-818-514-0038**
(Ext. 1)
Monday - Friday / 9am to 6pm

FIND US :

www.YourMusicConsultant.com
30721 Russell Ranch Road Suite 140 Westlake Village, USA
Email : info@yourmusicconsultant.com

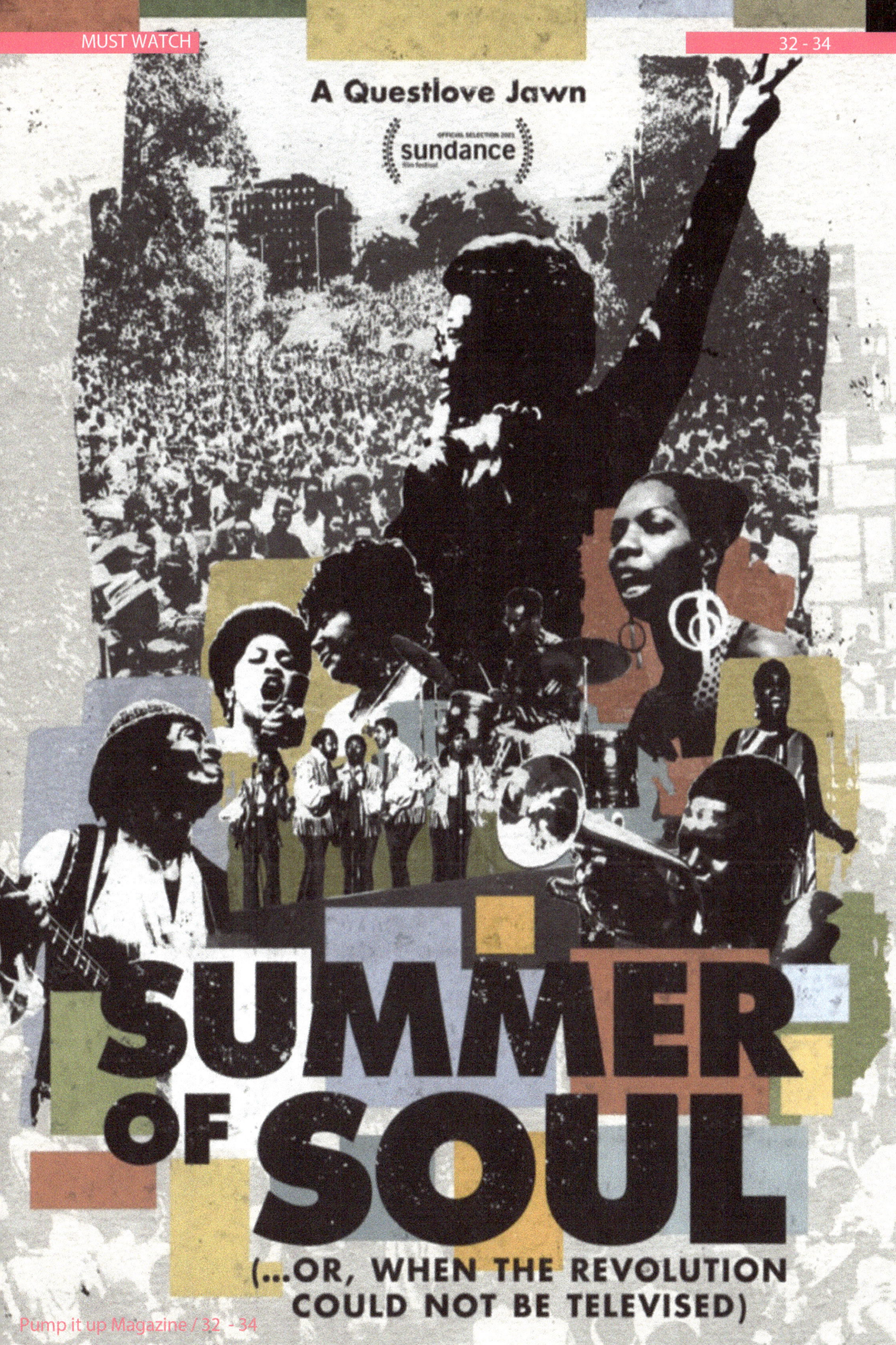

AWARENESS

WORLD ENVIRONMENT DAY

Celebrate World Environment Day by making a few easy changes the Earth will appreciate. In its simplest form, it's a day for people to step back, take a deep breath and appreciate Earth in all its splendor. But for many people Earth Day holds the potential to ignite broad environmental action.

As an internationally recognized holiday, World Environment Day is guaranteed to attract the attention of an enormous amount of people. So figuring out how to harness and activate that attention toward sustained action is something activists work hard on.

1) START COMPOSTING

Live video posts are shown in a user's newsfeed with the volume muted by default. And since Facebook users typically scroll quickly through their feed, it's a risk your video will get lost in the crowd. It's therefore a good idea to include the occasional use of text in your lower thirds to provide a snapshot of what the video is all about and attract the attention of potential viewers.

All you have to do is create a compost pile in your backyard or, if you're a city slicker, store all your vegetable, fruit, and other natural scraps in a plastic bag in your freezer and then dump it when full at a compost collecting place.

2) PLANT A GARDEN

Plant some flowers and get a beautifully fragrant garden. And then plant some vegetables and get all the produce you need. Here's a guide to starting a garden.

3) BUY A TREE CERTIFICATE

Trees are amazing. But humans relentlessly chop and burn them down. So this Earth Day buy a certificate from Stand for Trees to protect a batch of trees somewhere in the world that's at risk of deforestation.

4) BECOME A BETTER GROCERY SHOPPER

First, get a reusable grocery bag to limit all the plastic produced in the world.

Then try to buy fresh foods that you can carry in reusable containers. For example, fresh fruits and vegetables don't come prepackaged. Also, nuts, lentils, coffee beans and many other dry goods can generally be purchased from bulk containers. By using reusable containers, you're further reducing the amount of plastic in the world.

Finally, try to buy local, ethical and environmentally sustainable products. If you can't go local, go ethical and sustainable.

The Earth is a truly marvelous place that provides all of us with life. As humans, we can surely do a better job taking care of it.

www.ingramcontent.com/pod-product-compliance
Lightning Source LLC
Chambersburg PA
CBHW051810010526
44118CB00024BA/2822